REFLECTION ON AN EIGHTY YEAR JOURNEY
APRIL 1939 – AUGUST 2019

GRAEME RATTEN

First published by Busybird Publishing 2022

Copyright © 2022 Graeme Ratten

ISBN: 978-1-922691-50-7

This work is copyright. Apart from any use permitted under the *Copyright Act 1968*, no part of this publication may be reproduced, stored in a retrieval system or transmitted in any form or by any means, electronic, mechanical, photocopying, recording or otherwise, without the prior written permission of Graeme Ratten.

The information in this book is based on the author's experiences and opinions. The author and publisher disclaim responsibility for any adverse consequences, which may result from use of the information contained herein. Permission to use any external content has been sought by the author. Any breaches will be rectified in further editions of the book.

Cover Image: Graeme Ratten

Cover design: Busybird Publishing

Layout and typesetting: Busybird Publishing

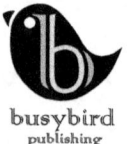

Busybird Publishing
2/118 Para Road
Montmorency, Victoria
Australia 3094
www.busybird.com.au

For Bev –

Who I have known for 70 years.
Who I have loved for 65 years.
To whom I have been married for 55 years.

We can only grow in proportion to what we give of ourselves, freely, in a genuine non-profit making sort of way.

"The Far Side of the Sky"
(Maslyn Williams)

CONTENTS

INTRODUCTION	1
FAMILY BACKGROUND	3
A JOURNEY THROUGH THE GENERATIONS	9
EARLY DAYS	14
SCHOOL DAYS	20
THE UNDERGRADUATE MEDICAL COURSE	28
POSTGRADUATE TRAINING	36
A CAREER IN OBSTETRICS AND GYNAECOLOGY	56
SOME CLINICAL PROBLEMS	71
JOURNEY IN FARMING	77
JOURNEY IN SPORT	82
JOURNEY IN MOTORING	85
JOURNEY IN FINANCE	89
JOURNEY IN RELIGION	92
JOURNEY WITH FAMILY	99
JOURNEY IN RETIREMENT	114
REFLECTION	127

INTRODUCTION

When one examines the books displayed under the heading *Biography* in the local library or in a bookstore it is evident that the majority relate to people commonly in the public eye: entertainers, politicians, scientists, and sports people. Autobiographies are even more limited, the majority relating to sporting heroes and politicians, commonly highlighting a small part of the subject's life deemed to be important or interesting, often ghost written, frequently released just prior to Christmas and containing some contentious material to gain media attention and publicity, thereby stimulating sales.

This book has been written for other reasons. Like many 80-year-olds I have some concern about the possibility of developing dementia, this concern being fostered by the fact that my paternal grandmother and my father's sister both suffered from this condition.

To minimise this risk one can follow the advice to exercise and to eat sensibly in order to reduce the likelihood of developing diabetes and hypertension, and, if indicated, to take statins to control cholesterol levels and aspirin to promote blood circulation. Mental activity such as reading newspapers and other informative literature, keeping abreast of current affairs, and solving Sudoku and crossword puzzles is thought to be important in reducing the risk as is promoting interpersonal relationships with a wide range of people. Generating literature is a step up from reading as a mental exercise and it is for this reason that I have been stimulated to write this account of my life.

Life has often been described as a journey; a journey which commences in the delivery room, and which concludes at the funeral parlour and many have observed, correctly, that the journey is more important than the ultimate destination. I prefer to think of life as a series of journeys, some such as childhood, adulthood, retirement, and old age defined by time; others such as occupation, hobbies and religion defined by function. Each of these journeys may impact on, or be affected by, other journeys that have been taken in the past or which are being undertaken concurrently.

To add interest to this record of a somewhat unremarkable journey I will endeavour, where appropriate, to note and comment on some of the amazing changes that have occurred in society during a lifetime of 80 years.

FAMILY BACKGROUND

The relative importance of 'nature' and 'nurture' in influencing what sort of person we become as we mature has been debated endlessly. A cursory glance at some individuals and their parents is all that is necessary to decide that genetics is important in shaping our physical characteristics. It is more difficult to assess whether our mental and psychic attributes are mainly inherited or mainly learned.

To provide some background information, it is appropriate to briefly consider my family history.

~~~

My paternal great-great-grandfather, Thomas Ratten (1795-1865), son of John Ratten and Elizabeth Smeathe, was born in Kennington, Kent, England. A farmer, he married Harriet Mummery and they travelled with six of their nine children to Australia as assisted passengers on the 327-ton barque *Sarah*, arriving in Melbourne in the Port Phillip district of the Colony of New South Wales on 1st January 1842. This was only six and a half years after John Batman had, in June 1835, signed a treaty with the elders of the Wurundjeri aborigines to acquire land in the area and noted that it was the place for a village. Governor Richard Bourke, in September 1837, visited the site and called it Melbourne, supplanting the previous name of Bearbrass which was a mis-rendering of the Wurundjeri term of Birrarung (River of Mists) previously used to describe the area. Melbourne was incorporated as a town in August 1842 eight months after Thomas Ratten and his family arrived, and in June 1887 was declared to be a city.

Two of Thomas and Harriet's children had died and the eldest, aged 22 years, elected to remain in England. Thomas purchased land in Hawthorn, developed a market garden and sold fresh vegetables. Elm cottage, the first commercial building in the area, and a family home were built on the corner of Power Street and Riversdale Road.

Great-grandfather Richard Ratten (1832-1879), seventh child of Thomas and Harriet, was nine years old when they arrived in Australia. He became a carpenter and builder and erected dwellings in Kew. In 1851, he and his brother Thomas travelled to the Bendigo gold fields, were successful, and upon return purchased land fronting Cotham Road, Kew. In 1852 Richard married Fanny Bird and they produced ten children, two of whom died in infancy.

Grandfather Ernest Spurgeon Ratten (1871-1928), eighth child of Richard and Fanny, held a management position with, and was ultimately managing director of, Parker and Bird timber merchants. Ernest married Florence Amelia Chapman in 1907, built a home on the corner of Florence Avenue and Cotham Road, Kew, and called it *Kennington* after his grandfather's birthplace. It was here that his two children were born.

My father Kenneth Ernest Ratten (1908-1975), eldest child of Ernest and Florence, studied medicine at the University of Melbourne. Following four years of postgraduate training he purchased a general practice at 4 Blyth Street, Brunswick in 1938 and worked there until his death in 1975.

~~~

My maternal great-great-grandfather John Daniel Manning (1789-1871) was born at Olney, Buckinghamshire, England, son of John Manning (1761-1829) of Newton, Blossomville, Buckinghamshire and Sussanah Hooten of Ravenstone, Buckinghamshire. John Daniel farmed a rented property while his father John farmed his own land. He married Eliza Andrews in 1812 and they had a large family of 12 children, ten of whom survived to adulthood.

Great grandfather George Manning (1826-1881), eighth child of John Daniel and Eliza, migrated to Australia travelling on the ship *Rajah* and disembarked at the colony of South Australia in 1850. Eighteen months later he travelled to the Victorian goldfields where he must have been successful as he returned to England in 1857 and married Mary Anne Rice Stainer of Margate, Kent. The newlyweds sailed to the colony of Victoria and their first child was born in Oakleigh in 1858. They lived in various country towns until George purchased land at Harston near Tatura. George died at the age of 55 leaving Mary Anne with eight children between the ages of eight and 22 years.

Grandfather Arthur Manning (1864-1915), eighth child of George and Mary Anne, farmed in the Tatura district with his brother Victor. Arthur purchased more property in the Waranga Basin region. He married Elizabeth Marshall Davidson and they produced five children.

My mother Dorothy Helen (nee Manning, 1910-1990) was the fourth child of Arthur and Elizabeth. She trained as a kindergarten teacher and married my father Kenneth Ernest Ratten on 25th August 1937.

~~~

Interestingly there are considerable similarities between the two families. Both came from shires in the south of England adjacent to London, Kent and Buckinghamshire. Both had a farming background.

The family members who migrated to Australia did so in the middle of the 19th Century, undoubtedly seeking a better future for themselves and their descendants. In the early 1800's eighty percent of cultivated land in England was owned by the aristocracy and gentry who lived on the rents derived by leasing their land to others and it was uncommon for a farmer to own freehold land. There were good reports coming back to England from Australia and people with farming and trade skills were encouraged to emigrate to Australia where there was opportunity to acquire freehold land in the colonies. Indeed, financial incentives were offered in the way of assisted passages to attract them.

Members of each family travelled to the Victorian goldfields, and each had some success.

A detailed family history has been compiled for each family (1-5) and perusal of these documents indicates that members of both families show the traits of conservatism and of a well-developed work ethic. Both families were heavily involved with their local church and members of both families made significant contributions to organisations such as schools, local government, and service organisations. These traits of conservatism and of voluntary contribution to church and community were prominent in my parents.

My father Kenneth Ernest Ratten spent his working life in general practice in Brunswick. Initially he was a solo practitioner permanently on call as night and weekend locum services were unknown during the war years. After eight years he was joined by partners as the practice grew in size and doctors returned from war duties. Ken was not a member of the armed forces but was awarded the rank of Honorary Captain for his work of medically assessing potential recruits.

Ken had an active association with the Baptist Church, initially at Kew where he served as secretary to the Intermediate section of the Sunday School, then at Coburg where he served as a Deacon. Other positions he held included council member of the Victorian Baptist Theological College (Whitley College) where he also acted as medical officer, member of the Council of Carey Baptist Grammar School and member of the Brunswick Rotary Club.

Ken was a calm, thoughtful and honest person. I had a very close relationship with him and there is no doubt that he was a significant role model for me particularly in the areas of work ethic and choice of vocation. There were however areas in which we differed markedly. I recall that he used to replace his car every two or three years, was quick to try new technologies, had his suits tailor made and purchased most of his other clothes from Henry Bucks, an up-market men's outfitter. These extravagances influenced me; I have kept most cars I have owned for around ten years, have mostly worn suits made by Fletcher Jones and purchased my other clothes on special. My wife says I only purchase technological items when they are going out of fashion or have been superseded.

Many medical practitioners of Ken's era purchased farms because of an interest in the land and a somewhat dubious taxation advantage. Ken acquired a property at Nagambie in 1950. Initially covering 640 acres (one square mile) and located eight kilometres southeast of Nagambie. The property was enlarged over the years to 1,200 acres together with a 2-acre block in the town with a large Victorian house. This development was a major interest to him and his family and continued as a substantial interest to my family and for me.

Ken had little interest in the arts and little musical ability and his reading was mostly confined to newspapers and medical journals. I recall that someone gave him a copy of William L. Shirer's book *The Rise and Fall of the Third Reich*. He never progressed beyond page 20 but said it was a marvellous sedative and used it as such for many years. I too have little musical ability; indeed, am so challenged in this area that I was asked to leave the school choir. However, I do enjoy reading and books have played an important role in my life.

My mother Dorothy Helen Ratten was the linchpin of the family, coping with the irregular hours of a doctor in general practice, organisation of the home and of the medical practice during the seven years that the family lived at the surgery premises and in later years running two households, one in Coburg and one in Nagambie.

Dorothy was an active member of the Baptist Church. She was superintendent of the Beginners Department of the Sunday School at Kew and made a major contribution at Coburg where she was leader of the Young People's Social Club. She was actively involved with the Baptist Union of Victoria as council member, member of the Management Committee of Hedley Sutton Nursing Home, of Whitley Theological College and of Strathcona Baptist Girls Grammar School.

More interested in literature and the arts than Ken, she was responsible for nurturing my interest in reading, both prose and poetry. Dorothy was a stickler for appropriate behaviour and good manners and as a result I still try to be meticulous about such things as opening doors for ladies and walking on the kerbside of the footpath.

Dorothy and Ken had a close relationship with our four children. They frequently took them to Nagambie for weekends when work commitments precluded Bev and I from leaving Melbourne and looked after them for longer times when we attended medical conferences. Following Ken's death in 1975, Bev and I and the children moved into the family home in East Ivanhoe and Dorothy moved to live in the house directly behind which fortuitously came onto the market at that time. This marvellous arrangement enabled her to spend much time with her grandchildren and, as she aged and became frail, we were able to offer her much support.

References below refer to text on Pg 6

1. Phyllis D. Vimpani, The Birds of Barrington and Beyond, Book 1, 1994
2. Phyllis D. Vimpani, The Birds of Barrington and Beyond, Book 2, 1994
3. Rosamond Barber, The Rattens
4. Rosamond Barber, The Pioneer Rattens of Two Continents, 1984
5. Marion Lofthouse, The Mannings Way of Life, 1989

A JOURNEY THROUGH THE GENERATIONS

Wikipedia defines a generation as 'all the people born and living at about the same time and who show similar characteristics'.

Traditionally a biological definition has been used to measure the time length of a generation, this being the average interval of time between the birth of parents and the birth of their offspring, say 20 to 25 years. This time length was satisfactory in the distant past but is irrelevant today because cohorts are changing so rapidly in response to new technologies, changes in study and career options and shifting society values. Today, a sociological definition is used rather than a biological one; a generation is a 'cohort of people born within a span of time who share a comparable age and lifestyle and who are shaped by the events, trends and developments which occurred during that span of time'. A century ago people tended to resemble their parents and the Jesuit saying 'give me a child till he is seven and I will show you the man' was reasonably accurate. However, in the last fifty years people have been moulded by the times they live in rather than by their parents.

~~~

In the 118 years since Federation sociologists recognise seven different generations in Australia.

My parents, born in 1908 and 1910 were part of the **Federation Generation** (1900-1924). This group experienced the pride of nationhood then were greatly affected by World War One and the following Great Depression. Some fought in two world wars and then experienced the post-World War Two economic boom, which changed society from relative austerity to relative plenty. They had great pride in their country, a strong work ethic, firm ties to Britain and loyalty to their spouses and to their employers.

I was born in 1939 during the Builders Generation (1925-1945) sometimes called the Silent, Conservative or Lucky Generation. Born in the crises of the Great Depression and World War Two but too young to really understand the problems they caused, this group were young adults during the post-World War Two boom with its years of relative comfort. Economically better off than their parents, they showed a similar loyalty to their spouses, their bosses and their country.

The **Baby Boomers** (1946-1964) have also been called the Stress, Me, Happy, Beatnik, TV and Disco Generation. Born during a time of economic growth, prosperity, full employment, free tertiary education and relatively low housing costs they are a generation who 'had it all'. They enjoyed increased freedom and better economic conditions than their parents and tended to be self-obsessed.

All our children – Kevin 1965, Andrew 1966, Janine 1968, and Nicola 1971 – were born in **Generation X** (1965 to 1977) sometimes called the Post-Boomers, Slackers, Whiners or Latch-Key Kids Generation. This generation shows similar characteristics to the Baby Boomers but live in an era not quite as economically favourable. They are sometimes described as having less loyalty to their spouses and employers with a tendency to a higher divorce rate and several changes of career as they seek greener pastures. Fortunately, our children do not show these traits and are blessed with stable personalities and a strong work ethic.

Generation Y (1978-1995) are also called the Millennial, Dot.com. or Kippers (that is Kids in Parents Pockets Eroding Retirement Savings) Generation. They are characterised by sociologists as a cohort who are inherently lazy with a limited attention span, unwilling to commit to binding relationships and with a relaxed moral code and high divorce rate. Addicted to computers they demand instant gratification and tend to be unrealistic and to want the easy option. Two of our grandchildren Larissa and Katelyn (1995) belong to this generation.

Generation Z (1996-2009) is sometimes called the iGeneration or the Gamers, and eight of our grandchildren belong to this cohort – Tom 1996, Sarah and Kane 1997, Kelly 1998, Stephanie and Joel 1999, Mitchell 2001 and Emily 2002. Members of this generation have an increased focus on formal education and spend much time on screens and digital devices. Their parents place high priority on education, homework, and coaching. This group tend to be sedentary and spend much time indoors and tend to be overweight. They are taller than their parents and much taller than their grandparents. They are the first generation to be fully global by connection through digital devices and engaging through social media. They have seen the development of Google (1997) Facebook and Twitter (2006), the iPhone (2007) and the iPad (2010). It is predicted that 50% will obtain a University degree compared 10% of Builders, 20% of Baby Boomers, 25% of Generation X and 33% of Generation Y.

Generation Alpha (2010+) is the first generation to be fully shaped in the 21st Century and the first generation who will see the 22nd century. They are being raised in a world of iPhones and screens.

~ ~ ~

Examination of the characteristics of these generations, as noted by sociologists, indicates there to be a gradual, but accelerating, trend away from conservatism, pride in nationhood, ties with Britain and loyalty to employer and spouse, together with a leaning towards self-centredness. There has been a change from relative austerity to relative plenty with better economic conditions and a higher standard of living. People have become better educated and their expectations about income and lifestyle have elevated. Travel and communication are much easier, better and cheaper and hours of work are much reduced. Somewhat paradoxically people tend to have become more sedentary and physically less able although, with better diet and medical care, longevity has increased. Levels of stress and of emotional insecurity seem to have increased.

~~~

It is interesting to reflect briefly on some of the changes in society and lifestyle that have occurred during the journey through the generations. Many of today's Z and Alpha Generation members have great difficulty in relating to some aspects of life in the Builders Generation.

I can recall my mother having to produce coupons to purchase food and clothing during the time of rationing of such items which occurred during and immediately following World War Two. All such purchases were made with cash as credit cards were not introduced until 1974. In some stores the shop attendant sent the record of purchase with the customer's cash by way of a container propelled along a wire to a central area where the sale was confirmed, and the appropriate change sent back by return container.

We received daily deliveries of milk and bread, both transported in a horse-drawn cart. The morning and evening newspapers were delivered by a paper boy and we received twice daily mail deliveries, the postman blowing a whistle as he placed the mail in the letterbox to notify the householder of the delivery.

There has been a quantum change in the type of food eaten by Australians. In the 1940's and 1950's the usual main meal (dinner) was grilled or roasted lamb or mutton with three vegetables, mashed potato, carrots and peas or beans. Fish and beef were occasionally eaten and on special occasions roast chicken or Shepherd's pie. Dessert was invariably tinned fruit served with ice cream, rice pudding or junket. Tea was the standard drink as coffee was invariably of poor quality.

School lunches were sandwiches, the filling being cold meat, Vegemite, jam, cheese, honey or, on special occasions, baked beans. In 1951 a Federal Government initiative for free milk was introduced into schools. The milk was not refrigerated and in summer was frequently unpalatable by lunch time.

The only take-away meals we enjoyed were occasional fried battered fish and chips. Pizza was unknown and the only spaghetti came in cans. There were few cafes and restaurants and

I cannot recall ever eating outside the home as a child and rarely as a teenager.

We have much to thank our post-war migrants for, in expanding and refining our diet.

Television was introduced into Melbourne in 1956 in time for the Melbourne Olympic Games. Initial uptake into homes was slow and large crowds gathered outside electrical stores to view this wonderful innovation. Our family obtained a set in 1958. Prior to this home entertainment was centred on the radio, there being the ABC and around four commercial stations, reading, board games and conversation. Picture theatres were popular, with local cinemas playing a program for children every Saturday afternoon.

Sport was played extensively, more so than today. Many attended the Victorian Football League matches on Saturday afternoon when two games were played, the Reserves commencing at midday followed by the Firsts. The Victorian Football Association matches were also well patronised. Interstate cricket matches, the Sheffield Shield, drew large crowds to the Melbourne Cricket Ground in summer, particularly if the match was between Victoria and New South Wales. The Test matches between Australia and England occurred every four years and were heavily patronised. Other sporting activities such horse racing at Caulfield and Flemington Racecourses, cycling at the velodrome, boxing and wrestling at Festival Hall drew large crowds. The introduction of television led to a drop in attendance at these sporting functions and to the cinema.

EARLY DAYS

In 1939 there were two events which had a huge impact on the people of Victoria.

On Friday 13th January (Black Friday) a fierce firestorm swept over the state, burning 2 million hectares of land, destroying 3,700 buildings including 1,300 homes and causing the death of 71 persons.

On Sunday 3rd September Prime Minister R.G. Menzies announced that in consequence of the persistence of Germany in her invasion of Poland, Great Britain had declared war upon her and that, as a result, Australia was also at war. During the six years of World War Two 993,000 Australians served in the armed forces and 27,073 were killed in action or died as a result of injuries sustained during the war.

It was midway between these two calamitous events that, on 22nd April, I was born at the Jessie McPherson Hospital, Melbourne.

The birth was not an easy one. My mother was in labour for three days following a pregnancy in which the only problem had been failure of the baby's head to enter her pelvis as full-term approached. In hindsight this was due to a posterior position of the foetal head, a complication which occurs in 10-15% of first pregnancies. It is frequently associated with a long slow painful labour and is nowadays treated with an epidural anaesthetic and syntocinon stimulation of uterine contractions, neither of which were available in 1939, and often requires Caesarean delivery. In the pre-antibiotic days of 1939 when anaesthetic and resuscitation techniques were unsophisticated, Caesarean section was regarded as a dangerous procedure and was performed infrequently. The Caesarean delivery rate was less than 3% in 1939 compared to greater than 30% in 2019 and the current dictum of never allowing the sun to set twice on a labouring woman did not apply. My mother's doctor, a general practitioner contemporary of my father, waited patiently until eventually a state was reached where vaginal delivery was possible. Doctor John Green, a prominent Melbourne obstetrician, attended and performed a difficult midforceps delivery under open ether anaesthesia. Delivery was achieved but mother and baby were so traumatized that they barely saw each other for three days. Eventually all was well although my mother did require a major pelvic repair operation in later life.

My father conducted a single-man general practice at 4 Blyth Street, Brunswick, and for the first seven years of my life we lived at the surgery. This was not an ideal venue for child-raising. There were two bedrooms, a small kitchen, a bathroom, and a tiny backyard with no children's play facilities. The remainder of the house was devoted to the medical practice. The patient's waiting room served as our sitting room in the evenings. There were major potential hazards for a young child in the form of sharp instruments, needles and dangerous drugs. There was also the need for peace and quietness. In those days there were no night-time or weekend locum services and the sole practitioner was on call all the time. Although there was a full-time receptionist/nurse there was need, at times, for my mother to act in that role. Child-minding and kindergarten facilities were not available in the 1940s.

Born before availability of immunization against the common childhood infectious diseases and living at the surgery, which would have been a hot bed of infection, I suffered from measles, mumps, rubella and chicken pox in the early years; fortunately, they were all mild cases without complications. More important were frequent colds which often led to fairly severe acute bronchitis. In the pre-antibiotic era this was treated with frequent applications of Vicks VapoRub to my chest and inhalation of steam containing Vicks. These attacks of bronchitis became so severe that my parents briefly considered moving to a warmer climate in Mildura but fortunately the problem lessened as I became older.

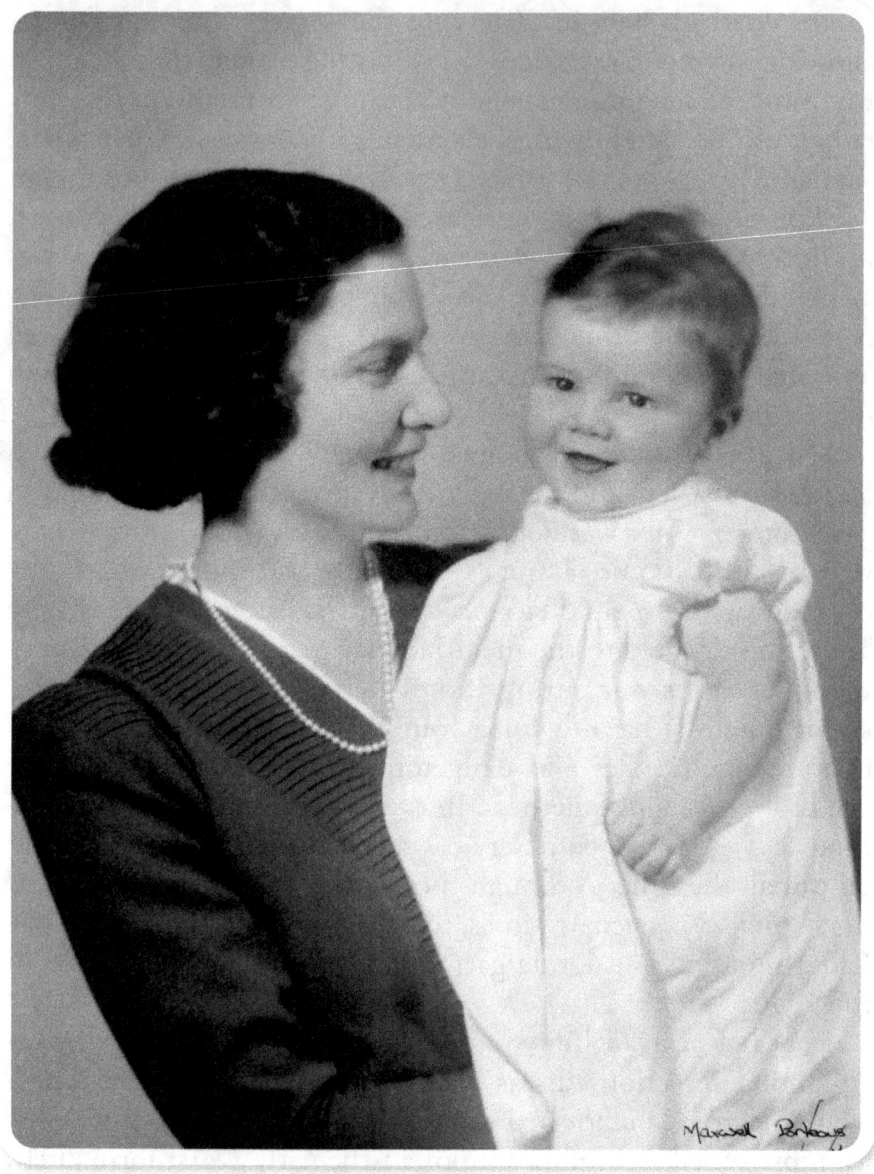

I have little memory of the first five years of life but do recall that I spent a great deal of time in the house next door where three maiden ladies, the Harrison sisters, lived with their brother who suffered a moderate degree of cerebral palsy. They became pseudo-aunts and taught me to read and write, probably as a way of entertaining me, with the result that I was quite literate by the time I commenced school.

Our social life was constrained by my father's work commitments and holidays were rare because of difficulty in obtaining locum medical cover during the war years. I do not recall having much contact with other children or with other family members. My paternal grandparents and maternal grandfather were no longer alive and of my five aunts and four uncles, four lived far from Melbourne and one spent most of World War Two overseas as a Padre with the Australian army. We did regularly visit my maternal grandmother who lived in Kew. One form of entertainment I do recall were occasional visits to the Times Theatrette in Bourke Street, Melbourne which showed an endlessly repeating one hour program of news interspersed with occasional cartoons. There was, of course, no television and

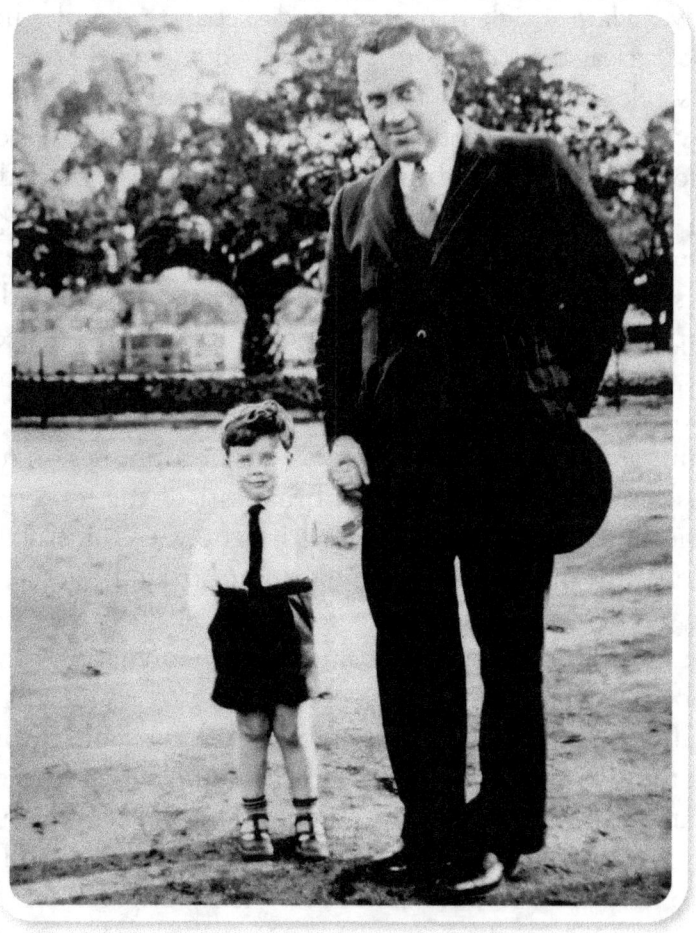

home entertainment was centred on books, board games and the radio.

In 1946 the family, now four in number with the addition of Kathleen (now Kate) born in 1944, moved to a residence at 43 The Grove, Coburg. This was a large house with five bedrooms, two sitting rooms, a dining room, and an attic large enough to accommodate a full-size billiard table and an old dining table which was used for table tennis. The house was well appointed but as was common in those days there was only one internal toilet and the only heating was a small gas fire in the seldom used dining room, open fires in the sitting rooms and a kerosene heater in the kitchen. There was no air-conditioning nor ceiling fans. The garden was large with a lawn area which could accommodate a cricket pitch and there was room in the backyard for a fowl run. There was a large brick incinerator and a separate complex housing a two car garage, a tool room, a woodshed and an external toilet.

This relocation made an enormous difference to my life. I quickly struck up a friendship with Peter Stevenson who lived next door and this friendship endures to this day. We had room to play cricket and football, much to the detriment of the garden and the windows adjacent to the lawn area. Fortunately, Peter was responsible for most of the broken windows and his father, an accomplished tradesman, was able to rapidly effect the necessary repairs. If the weather was inclement, we played billiards or table tennis.

I built a crystal set and was able, with headphones on, to drift off to sleep listening to a relayed broadcast of the test cricket in England much to my mother's chagrin who was concerned that a thunderstorm might occur, and lightning strike the aerial.

A gardener came one day a fortnight to keep the extensive garden in order and to repair some of the depredation caused by the football. My only outdoor chores were to ensure that there was sufficient kindling and split firewood available during the winter months and to care for the fowls. I built a fowl-house in the backyard and we kept a dozen Rhode Island Reds and a number of Bantams; it was my responsibility to feed them, to collect the eggs, to keep the run clean and occasionally dispatch one for the oven. It is certain that wherever there are fowls there will be rats and mice. This upset my mother and my father procured a jar of strychnine with the idea of poisoning them. Second thoughts about the danger of this plan led to him abandoning it and the strychnine was locked away in a safe which he had used at the surgery to house dangerous drugs. It stayed there for 30 years and eventually became my problem when dealing with his estate. Strychnine is difficult to dispose of safely and after discussion I was able to prevail on Fairfield Infectious Diseases Hospital, who had a high temperature incinerator, to deal with it. They were reluctant to take it but acquiesced after I, tongue in cheek, threatened to flush it down the toilet.

My Christmas present in 1949 was a bicycle, a rather up-market model with three speed Sturmey-Archer gears. Having convinced my parents that I could ride it safely, it became my main form of transport. Traffic was light and Peter and I rode far and wide on our bikes. I recall travelling to Nagambie by train at the age of 14 years, unaccompanied, with my bike in the guard's van and riding from Nagambie to Tatura to visit my aunt and uncle at their farm.

As the years passed, I became successively involved in the academic and sporting aspects of school, the religious, social and sporting activities of the Coburg Baptist Church, our farm property at Nagambie and the study involved in achieving a medical degree.

Bev and I met at Sunday School when we were about ten years old, became an item in our mid-teens and eventually married after we had both completed our tertiary education, Bev in general nursing and midwifery and me in medicine. We both lived in our respective family homes until the time of our marriage.

SCHOOL DAYS

I commenced formal education in 1945 at the Teachers Training College Rural Practicing School, which was located on the corner of Swanston and Grattan Streets, Carlton in the grounds of the Teachers Training College. The school consisted of three classrooms, each with a permanent teacher, Mr Heffernan, Miss Coghlan and Mr Wade, and each having around 30 pupils distributed between Grades 1 and 8. Several times a year, education students planning to teach in single teacher rural schools came to practice their teaching skills under the watchful eye of the permanent staff. Pupils sat at two person desks arranged in four rows of four, each desk having a lift up lid and a cavity to store books and other equipment and each having two recessed inkwells to enable us to dip our steel-nibbed pens.

The teacher's time had to be divided among the eight grades and, as a result, we were set work to perform. When one had completed the assigned task we were encouraged to read books available from a small library kept at the rear of the classroom. I suspect that this was responsible in part for my enduring love of reading.

I was able to read and write quite well before starting school and, as a result, was quickly promoted to grade 2, the downside of this being that, for the rest of my school days, I was one year younger than my contemporaries, although, as a larger than average child, this did not matter.

The academic environment was highly competitive, and we all entered into the spelling and mental arithmetic competitions with gusto. Corporal punishment in the form of a leather strap to the hand was administered for major misdemeanours.

The Herald *Learn to Swim* campaign was active at the time and on infrequent occasions all children walked one kilometre to the Melbourne City Baths to receive swimming lessons and ultimately a Herald Certificate indicating that they could successfully swim 25 yards.

Initially my father drove me to school and mother would pick me up, but very soon I travelled by tram, a one penny fare from Blyth Street, Brunswick and a twopence fare from Moreland Road, Coburg.

Every Monday morning, weather permitting, we assembled outside the classrooms and, after a formal assembly, saluted the flag and sang the National Anthem before marching into school to the beat of a drum played by one of the students.

The primary school education I received in the Government system was excellent. Discipline was firm and we were encouraged to learn basic skills albeit in a somewhat competitive manner and were firmly encouraged to read widely. The biggest downside was the inability to play competitive sport because the small number of children of similar age precluded formation of a team. There was a concrete cricket wicket available for practice and a grassed area large enough to kick a football.

~~~

In 1949 I left the State School and continued my education at Carey Baptist Grammar School in Year 6, the senior Middle School form also called Senior Remove. Carey, in Kew, was far from our home in Coburg and I spent the first two years as a weekly boarder. Weekly boarders were a despised group, pitied by day boys as they did not have the advantage of home life and parents during the week and despised as wimps by full boarders as they did have the advantage of home life at weekends. Weekly boarders left the school on Friday afternoon and returned in time for Chapel at 7:00pm on Sunday.

I have many memories of the boarding house but the most vivid is the incredible cold in our dormitory. Four of the most junior boys slept in a passageway which linked the upper stories of two buildings, Urangeline the original building on the Carey site and Laycock House where the boarders slept on the first floor. We were separated from the elements only by canvas blinds. Meals were good and were taken in the boarders' dining room on the ground floor of Urangeline.

The evening meal was followed by prayers and then by homework when one had to stay for a standard time, in perfect silence, whether one had homework or not, supervised by the senior boarding school master Mr Les Trewin.

Boarders had to make their beds each morning and I can remember a few occasions when we were involved in washing and drying dishes because of an acute shortage of kitchen staff. My talent in bed making endures to this day but I am not encouraged in this area because of my inability to construct 'hospital corners' so beloved by nurses. Boarders used the time between cessation of lessons and dinner to play sport or to dig extensive and elaborate tunnels in the vacant land on the north aspect of the school. Chapel on Sunday night was taken by Headmaster Mr Stuart Hickman, and I can still remember some of the homilies that he delivered.

I became a day student in 1951 and travelled by tram from Coburg to Kew via the Melbourne Central Business District, a trip taking about one hour.

My academic performance at Carey was a little like the curate's egg, good in parts. Reviewing my term reports which my parents, for no good reason, kept show an even mixture of A's and B's with a smattering of C's and an occasional D. Comments by teachers were generally positive but there were a significant numbers of remarks such as 'disappointing' or 'can do better than this'.

My recollection of the standard of teaching we received at Carey is that it was somewhat variable:

- Headmaster Stuart Hickman who knew the name of all 400 boys at the school and who took some French lessons was admired by all.

- Senior Master Charles "Bunny" Gramlick taught Mathematics. He had a disconcerting technique of asking students if there were any problems in the text book they could not solve and having received a negative answer, which was usually because no-one had attempted any of the problems, started on new work.

- Rev. John Morley was Chaplain and taught Biology. In the first role he was admired, able to paint vivid word pictures to boys and young men about religious matters. I do not remember him as being a great success as Biology teacher.

- John Sykes was English teacher and coach of the First XI and did both jobs brilliantly. He had a curious habit of 'losing' his spectacles by pushing them up on his forehead, forgetting he had done this, and sending pupils from his class all over the school in search of them. John had a fixation about corsets – he would yell 'Get them off!' to any cricketer who was slow to pick up the ball at fielding practice.

- Brian Baird was Geography master and his somewhat laconic approach was admired by all who attended his classes.

- RH "Drak" Wilkinson taught Physics and Chemistry. He was bearded, drove an Alfa Romeo and eventually left Carey to take up a position as lecturer at Melbourne University, which was probably good for both institutions. He had a large fund of jokes, and I can remember one mid-winter day as we sat in the unheated classroom and complained about the cold he lit a bunsen burner on the front desk and proceeded to warm his hands.

- Norman Dobson was Social Studies master and had a vast collection of daily newspapers which the matriculation students raided and took to the prefect's common room to burn in the open fireplace. He was the most organised of our teachers and produced printed notes outlining the syllabus and the matters we needed to consider.

- Charles Bucknill was the French master. I did almost no study, scraped through the examination and dropped French as soon as I could, after year 10. Charlie and I were not the closest of friends and he was, I think, devastated when he came across my sons 25 years later who had the same attitude to French as I had.

Committed to making a career in Medicine it was necessary for me to ignore the humanities and concentrate on science subjects. I passed Year 12, then called Matriculation, in 1955 taking the subjects English Expression, Physics, Chemistry, Pure Mathematics and Calculus and Applied Mathematics. My marks were adequate for admission into the Medical Course at Melbourne University and for me to be awarded a Government Scholarship which would pay for University fees. For reasons I will discuss later I returned to school in 1956 taking and passing the subjects Physics, Chemistry, Calculus and Applied Mathematics, Biology, Geography and Social Studies. I enjoyed this year at school as with, no concern about passing Matriculation, I was able to be more involved in the sporting and non-academic aspects of school life.

I was appointed a school Prefect in 1955, a position which carried with it some honour and limited responsibility such as yard duty during the lunch break. Carrying more kudos was my election by the students in Steele House to the position of House Captain in my final year at Carey.

I was awarded several academic prizes during my time at Carey but the most notable was a half-scholarship won at an examination taken in Year 8 which my father donated back to the school to be used to make it possible for a boy from a financially deprived background to attend the school. I also gained first place in a statewide essay competition run by the Shell Company of Australia.

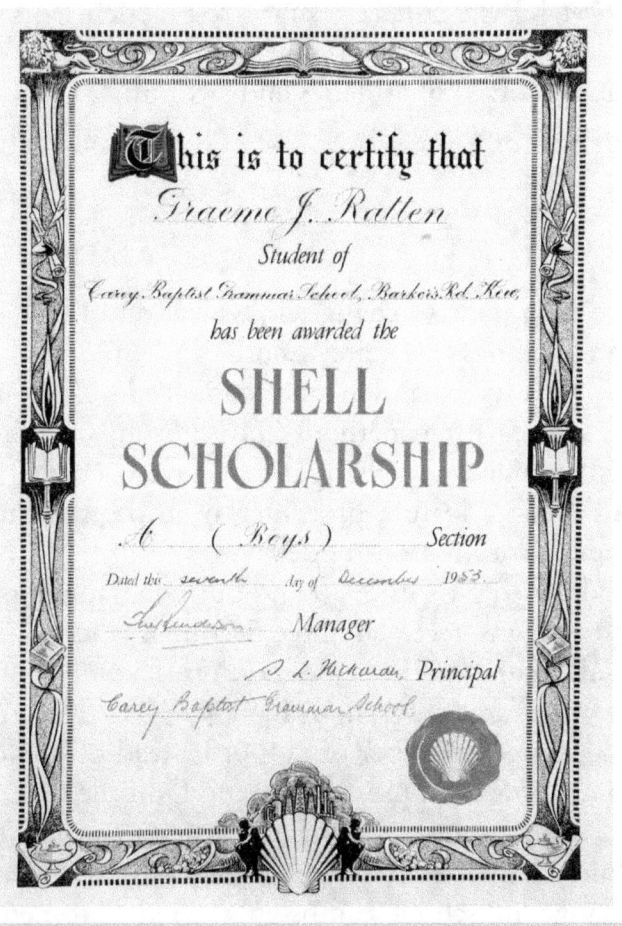

Sport was important at Carey and members of the First XI and the First XVIII were seen as heroes. There was internal competition between the four Houses, Moore, Steele, Sutton and Tranter and external competition against the other Associated Grammar Schools, Brighton, Camberwell, Caulfield, Haileybury and Trinity. I played cricket, football and tennis for Steele House and represented the school in the First XVIII and in the First XI in which I was opening bowler for three years and vice-captain in my final year.

I received a measure of notoriety for hooking a wayward delivery through an upstairs window of Laycock House, a building located some 30 metres beyond the boundary of the oval. Vivian Richards performed this feat 25 years later when the touring West Indian cricket team were practicing on the Carey oval.

I was not involved in athletics and swimming as I had no skill in these areas.

~~~

There have been massive changes in education in the last seventy years. The facilities at Carey, both academic and sporting, have been greatly expanded and enhanced. Computers have revolutionised teaching methods and the subjects available and the curriculae reflect the changes that have occurred in society. Music and Theatre feature prominently in the syllabus but one can rue the lack of interest in poetry.

Carey admitted girls in 1979 and our two daughters, together with our two sons received their Secondary School education there and all assure me that co-education is a positive thing. The number of pupils at the school has increased from 400 in my time to the current number of 2,400. Instead of one campus at Kew there are now campuses at Kew and Donvale with a sporting complex at Bulleen and a permanent school camp at Toonalook on the Ninety Mile Beach.

The change in school camps is a good barometer for the change in the education system. Each of our children spent four or five days in school camps on two occasions during their time in a Government primary school. During their secondary school education at Carey they attended camps in Year 7 at Toonalook, in Year 9 at Hattah Lakes, in Year 10 an Outward Bound camp at varying venues and a Humanities Camp in Year 11. Janine, who had four years of secondary school education at Strathcona prior to transferring to Carey, spent Year 9 at an off-main-campus venue at Tay Creggan. Bev attended each Humanities camp as a cook, leaving me with the other three children for the week. We lived on barbecues and frozen meals she had left for us. On her return she was always amazed by the disreputable state of the house, despite a cursory clean-up we performed on the day before her return. Most upsetting for her was the state of the kitchen which she described as grey in appearance with the original dishcloth and towels still in use.

Our grandchildren have had similar camp experiences. Indeed those attending a private school in Shepparton each had a two week 'Get to Know Melbourne' exercise and then a three week trip to either Borneo, Costa Rica or Indonesia. This contrasts with my experience in which the only off-campus activities were occasional visits, walking, to the local Council swimming pool and a one-day tour of the Shell Oil Refinery.

~~~

The overall impression that comes to mind when I think of school, as it was when I attended in the 1940's and 1950's, is that it was a time of good fellowship and minimal aggravation. We were encouraged to develop a social conscience and to be tolerant of people of different religions and social backgrounds. We were not spoon-fed but thrown on our own resources a great deal. This did prepare us for University in a way that gave us an advantage over students from some other schools.

THE UNDERGRADUATE MEDICAL COURSE

Although the results I obtained at the Matriculation Examination in 1955 at the age of 16 years were sufficient to gain entry to the medical course and to be awarded a Government Scholarship the Registrar of Melbourne University, Mr Marginson, stated that the University did not want me to start the course until I was 17 years old and that I should have another year at school and would then be assured of a place to commence in 1957. My father agreed to this and I had a second year in Matriculation, a year I thoroughly enjoyed, studying some different subjects.

I presented to the University to enrol at the end of 1956 to be told that, although I had passes in eight Matriculation subjects, my total score was now not good enough to enter the medical course, a situation which led to some robust discussion between my father and Mr Marginson. The University would not move from their position and it was finally agreed that I should do one year of a science course, Botany, Chemistry, Physics and Zoology, and that they would then consider allowing me to enter the second year of the medical course if my academic performance was satisfactory. I enjoyed the year, achieved third class honours in all subjects and accordingly was permitted to enter the second year of the medical course in 1958 to study Anatomy, Biochemistry and Physiology. Unfortunately, I failed in Biochemistry, the only examination I failed in my formal education, and had to repeat the year.

The first three years of the medical course, spent at the University of Melbourne, were devoted almost entirely to basic sciences with minimal patient contact while the second three years were spent at various teaching hospitals with only a few lectures at the University.

I studied Medicine and Surgery at the Royal Melbourne Hospital and spent 12 weeks at each of the Royal Children's Hospital and the Royal Women's Hospital. I found the clinical years to be far more interesting and stimulating than the pre-clinical years and enjoyed contact with patients and involvement in various practical procedures.

PRE-CLINICAL YEARS

The first two years of the six year course were devoted to studying the basic sciences, Biochemistry, Chemistry and Physics, followed by the more relevant Anatomy and Physiology. There were formal lectures given by Professors and Associate Professors in each of these subjects together with many hours devoted to practical work and less formal tutorials presided over by junior members of the relevant university departments.

In third year we continued to study Anatomy and also Histology, Microbiology and Bacteriology, Pathology and Therapeutics. The lectures and practical work were more disease-orientated and one at last had the feeling that the knowledge we were gaining was appropriate to the practice of medicine.

ROYAL MELBOURNE HOSPITAL

On our first day at the RMH, a hot day in mid-January, we were rostered to view a post-mortem examination. It was conducted by a jovial young pathologist who delighted in demonstrating his work in a small non-air-conditioned room with flair. The 40 students stood on platforms around the operating table. It was not long before some students were forced to leave because of nausea and faintness and, by the end of the procedure, only ten remained.

There were three teaching streams at RMH. Several times a week all 40 students attended a formal lecture given by one of the hospital's consultant doctors or by the Professor or a member of his department.

For hands-on clinical teaching we were divided into groups of five or six. Each group attended Outpatient Clinics where we were expected to take a medical history from a patient then examine them with one of the doctors working in the clinic, who would discuss the problem with the patient and the student. For inpatient teaching students were allotted three or four patients in one of the hospital's wards and were expected to visit them each day and be conversant with their management and progress. The ward registrar, usually a third-year trainee, would involve us in any procedures that might be performed on the patients and gave us informal tutorials.

Students were expected to accompany allotted patients to the operating theatre if they required surgery and were usually able to scrub and assist with the procedure. Once a week the senior consultant doctor for the ward would take students for a ward round of all patients and give a formal tutorial. This method of teaching certainly gave students the opportunity to develop their skills in communicating with and examining patients.

Students spent one month in the Emergency Department during which time they worked with the doctors who were assessing patients and, if appropriate, were involved in their treatment. Students sutured all minor lacerations under local anaesthesia, performed small skin grafts and procedures such as insertion of intravenous lines and passage of catheters and, rarely, lumbar punctures.

ROYAL CHILDRENS HOSPITAL

Our time at RCH, ten weeks in fifth year and two weeks in final year, was pleasant, no doubt partly due to the fact that the medical and nursing staff who work with children are, for the most part, pleasant, calm and tolerant – if not they would not be able to cope with the stresses involved in caring for their young patients.

Teaching of medical students was conducted in a similar fashion to the teaching at RMH with formal lectures given to the whole group of 40 students and small group involvement with patient contact in Inpatient, Outpatient and Emergency

Department areas with associated tutorials. One big difference from adult medicine was the amount of time spent in considering the large range in what is normal in children with respect to such basic matters as size, weight, development of motor and communication skills and other physical functions. Much attention was given to infant and toddler feeding. The small size of the patients precluded students from being involved in procedures such as surgical repair of minor lesions.

ROYAL WOMENS HOSPITAL

The same basic methods of teaching were employed at RWH as at RMH and RCH with one huge difference – students were required to be resident in the hospital for ten weeks in fifth year and two weeks in final year. This was necessary because much of the action in obstetrics, and therefore many of the learning opportunities, occured out of office hours.

Whilst lectures, clinics and ward rounds were attended during the day, students were required to be available at all times to be involved in births and other procedures in delivery suite and in the operating theatre and to attend impromptu tutorials given by consultant obstetricians who attended the hospital to deal with obstetric problems. Students were allotted to care for antenatal patients in the wards and had to be available to sit with them during their labour and to be involved in their delivery. Unlike the situation at RCH medical students at RWH enjoyed much practical involvements with patients. They were required personally to conduct 20 deliveries, including one forcep delivery, under the supervision of senior mid-wives or junior medical staff, and were available to suture the episiotomies which had been made to facilitate deliveries conducted by nursing students.

I found the time at RWH to be the most enjoyable part of the medical course, partly because of the extensive practical involvement and also because the majority of the patients were healthy young women of a similar age to the medical students and most were in hospital enjoying a happy experience. Of course there were some whose pregnancy did not end happily because of still-birth or congenital abnormality of the baby or whose gynaecological condition was not readily amenable to treatment; involvement with these patients gave us some insight into how to deal with unfavourable outcomes in medicine.

OTHER TEACHING VENUES

All students were required to attend short courses of lectures and demonstrations at Royal Victorian Eye and Ear Hospital and at Peter MacCallum Cancer Centre.

Some attended a ward round and tutorial held every Sunday morning at Prince Henry's Hospital conducted by a dynamic young surgeon who was considered to be an excellent teacher.

All students spent two weeks during fifth year in a General Medical Practice. Since the majority of graduates would eventually become family doctors, the University considered it to be important that students were exposed to the type of work such a career would entail. Students had to arrange this themselves and I spent the two weeks at Brunswick Medical Clinic with my father and his four partners.

EXAMINATIONS

Examinations were held in Anatomy, Biochemistry, Chemistry, Physics, Physiology, Microbiology and Pathology during the three pre-clinical years.

There were no further examinations until the end of final year. We then had examinations in Medicine, Surgery and Obstetrics and Gynaecology. There were two three-hour written papers in each subject, all essay questions as short answer as multiple choice questions had not yet become popular.

There were also two oral examinations in each subject. One was a long case requiring the candidate to take a history from the patient, perform a physical examination and then present the case to two examiners who would question him/her about management. The other involved questions from the examiner based around a series of patients who had readily visible lesions and occasionally x-rays. Candidates who did well in these examinations were invited to attend a further oral examination to assess whether they warranted an honours ranking.

I was fortunate to be invited to attend an honours oral in all three subjects and achieved third class honours in Surgery and in Obstetrics and Gynaecology and was ranked equal fourth among the 160 students who graduated in 1963.

Two incidents that occurred during the examinations I took are worthy of mention.

The oral examination in Anatomy in second year required candidates to rotate through six stations, each presided over by a lecturer from the Anatomy Department who asked questions about dissected specimens lying on the table. My second station contained various specimens of the upper limb and the examiner was a very stern Associate Professor. I successfully identified various tendons, muscles and nerves he pointed to then was asked to name the tendons visible in a dissection of the front of the wrist. I became disorientated and named them incorrectly – his response was to shout 'You bloody idiot!' in a voice loud enough to attract the attention of everyone in the room.

In the final clinical examination, the patient seen in the long case in each discipline was usually a person who had been admitted to the hospital because of a problem; it was, of course, an ordeal for the patient as well as the candidate. My patient in the long obstetric case was a lady who had been admitted in labour but whose labour had ceased. A pleasant lady with three children all born normally she did not seem to have any problem; however by the time I saw her labour had recommenced and she was having contractions every two or three minutes. I elicited her history and was performing a general examination when she suddenly gave a loud grunt and the baby appeared in the bed. I gingerly picked it up, being careful not to get my suit soiled, and called for help from the nursing staff. When I met the examiners their first question was 'What was the problem with your patient?' I replied that she was in labour. 'How do you know?' they asked. 'Because I delivered the baby!' They laughed heartily at this. Further questioning went well and I felt confident that I would receive a good mark.

CHANGES IN STUDENT TEACHING

There had been an explosion of knowledge in medicine, as in all other branches of science, during the last fifty years. Students have to achieve a dauntingly high score in the Victorian Certificate of Education to gain admission to the medical course. The course has been modified so that less emphasis is placed on basic sciences such as Physics, Chemistry and Anatomy but there is more emphasis on Physiology and the way in which the body functions or malfunctions.

Students now become involved with patient care early in the course rather than patient contact being restricted to the last three years. Importantly there is more emphasis on diagnosis and management of mental and emotional problems. In order to find time to fit this into the syllabus students spend less time studying Paediatrics and Obstetrics and Gynaecology.

Whilst students graduating today have a vastly greater theoretical knowledge than graduates of 55 years ago, they have less practical experience of minor surgery and procedures performed in the Emergency Department and in delivering babies.

Unlike the situation that pertained 55 years ago it is now mandatory for all graduates to work for a year as an intern in a public hospital and most complete several further years of post-graduate training during which time they obtain practical experience.

There have been major changes in the methods of assessing medical students. Fifty years ago written examination questions took the form of a few questions to be answered in essay form, thus assessing the students' depth of knowledge in a small number of areas. Today written examination papers are either multiple choice format or take the form of a larger number of short answer questions thus assessing knowledge over a wider range of topics.

Fifty years ago, clinical examinations required the candidate to interview an actual patient, take the history and examine them, present the case to the examiner and discuss the diagnosis and the management of the problem. Students taking the examination would see different patients presenting problems of varying complexity; the examiner had to allow for this when assessing the candidate's knowledge and skills. In order to overcome this difficulty, clinical examinations are now conducted differently; an artificial scenario is used so that all candidates face the same clinical problem, and the patient is replaced by a role player who gives a pre-arranged identical history to all candidates. The candidates are required to demonstrate how they would examine the patient and are then provided with an identical set of clinical signs. They discuss the diagnosis and management with the role-playing 'patient', the whole process being observed by the examiner. This method of assessment has the great advantage that all candidates face the same clinical problem, and it also allows the examiner to assess the candidate's ability to communicate with the patient.

POSTGRADUATE TRAINING

After successfully passing the final examination the Degrees of Bachelor of Medicine and Bachelor of Surgery, Melbourne were conferred at a ceremony held at Wilson Hall, University of Melbourne on 14th December 1963.

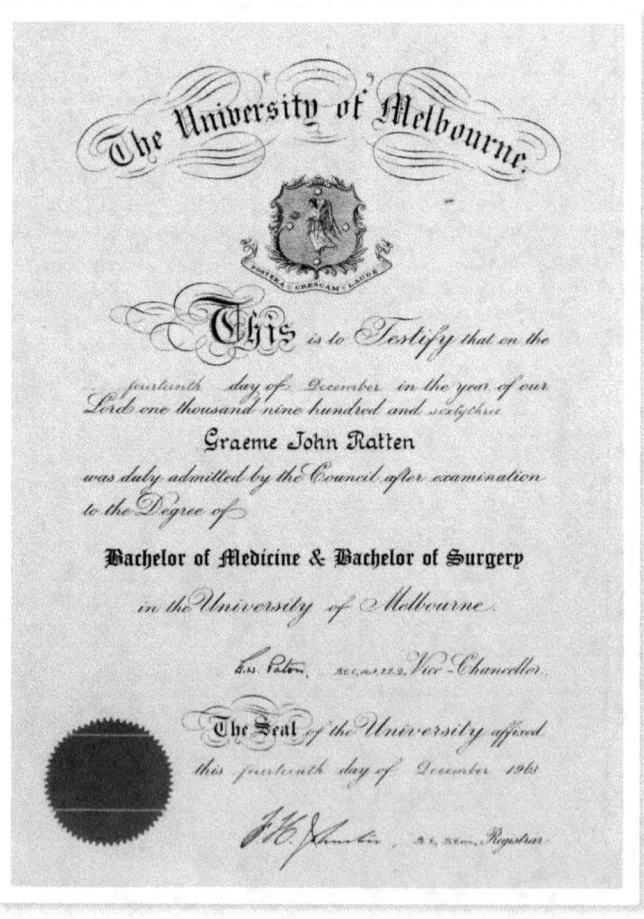

POSTGRADUATE TRAINING

I was registered as a legally qualified medical practitioner by the Medical Board of Victoria and my name was added to the Medical Register.

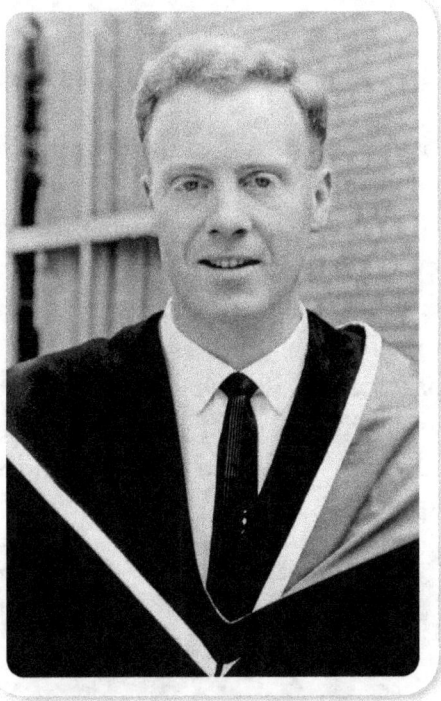

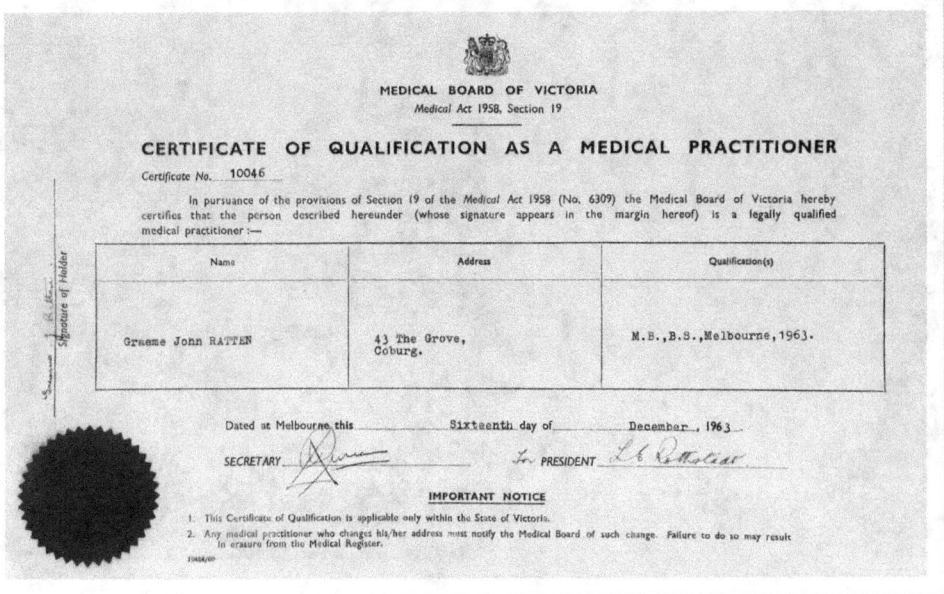

Graduates who wished to undergo further training had to apply for a position as Resident Medical Officer in a Victorian Public Hospital. Having achieved good marks in the final examination I was awarded my first choice.

ROYAL MELBOURNE HOSPITAL

I commenced postgraduate training as a Junior Resident Medical Officer (RMO) at RMH in mid-January 1964, three weeks after Bev and I were married. The 12-month program entailed three months in a general medical ward, three in a general surgical ward, two in the Emergency Department, two at Fairfield Infectious Diseases Hospital and one month in each of the Cardiac and Anaesthetic Departments. The average time rostered on duty was 120 hours per week with time off duty being one afternoon, two evenings and nights per week and every second weekend.

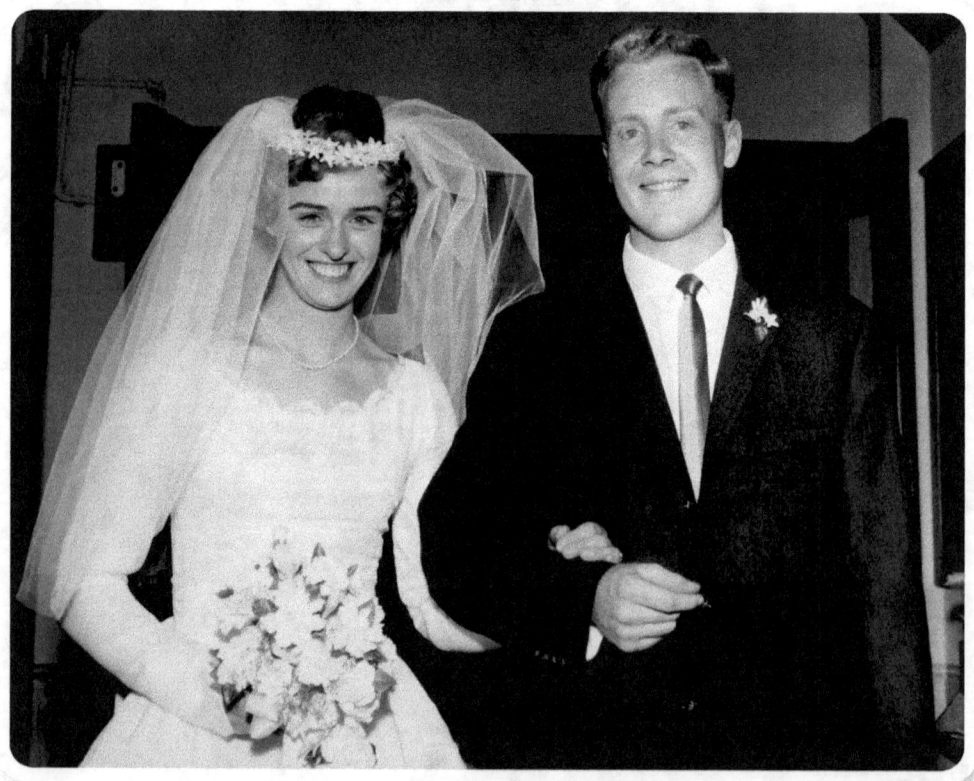

The days and evenings were extremely busy, the nights less so and Bev used to sleep at the hospital often where we would share a single bed.

RMO's are in many ways rather like apprentices in a trade such as building or plumbing. They received some formal instruction but most of their theoretical knowledge and practical skills are gained by assisting a skilled and experienced senior person or working under close supervision. They are also, like trade apprentices, paid a meagre salary. The salary I received of 19 Pounds (38 Dollars) per week was marginally greater than the basic wage for adult males in Victoria of $30.70. However, in consequence of the long hours we worked the salary equated to a pay rate of 31 cents per hour rostered on duty.

There was an enormous opportunity to increase my theoretical knowledge and to learn new practical skills although the former was somewhat inhibited by chronic tiredness. The senior consultant doctors and senior Resident Medical Officers were very supportive and keen to impart their knowledge to RMO's who, in turn, were expected to demonstrate basic skills such as suture of wounds and insertion of intravenous lines to medical students. Meals were often skipped because of work pressure and I lost six kilograms weight in the first three months – due to missing meals, not due to Bev's cooking.

The ward duties of an RMO included clerking (taking the history from, examining and documenting) all patients on admission, doing a full round of all 30 inpatients each day and documenting their progress, being available to do a ward round with the registrar each day and with the senior consultant doctor twice a week. We met with ancillary staff such as Social Workers and Physiotherapists to plan patient's ongoing care and spoke to patient's relatives to appraise them of progress. A letter had to be written to the patient's local doctor when they were discharged from hospital.

Whilst we attained much practice in dealing with injuries and lacerations in the Emergency Department there was great competition for surgical cases needing to be dealt with in the Operating Theatre and most RMO's managed to perform a couple of appendectomies during the year. Conversely we were given a great deal of responsibility by the Anaesthetic Department and were entrusted to administer anaesthesia for a variety of surgical procedures with minimal supervision.

The term at Fairfield Infectious Diseases Hospital was notable for several reasons; the work load was lighter and the pace less frenetic, although we did have to do many lumbar punctures, particularly when rostered for an overnight shift – which happened three times a week; and the gentlemanly way in which the medical staff were organised with a roast meal for lunch most days, served on fine china.

During the term with the Cardiac Department, RMO's were deputised to attempt resuscitation of patients in the ward who suffered an unexpected cardiac arrest. Responding to a Code Call on the hospital PA system, we proceeded with haste to the ward taking with us the crash cart which contained all the drugs which might be needed, an electrocardiograph machine and a defibrillator. Regrettably successful resuscitation was rare, largely because most of the patients we were called to were of advanced years and suffering from advanced disease.

This year saw enormous changes in my life. Previously I had been in an organised world in which I lived at home, cared for by my parents, and despite having to spend time studying, was able to play sport and socialise with friends from school and church and, in general, lead a pleasant relaxed stress-free life. I had entered a disorganised world in which working hours were long leading to chronic fatigue, major decisions had to be made which could have an impact on other people's lives and wellbeing, bereaved relatives had to be counselled and there was no time for sport and little for socialising. Importantly my medical knowledge had increased and there had been great improvement in my skills in clinical assessment of patients, in performing practical procedures and in communicating with patients and their relatives; all of which gave me great satisfaction and confidence that I was going to enjoy my career in medicine.

ROYAL CHILDRENS HOSPITAL

In February 1965, after two weeks holiday, I commenced work as an RMO at RCH, spending three months in a general medical ward, three in a general surgical ward, four in the Emergency Department and two in the Respiratory Unit which treated neonates and young children with respiratory disorders such as croup and bronchiolitis.

The workload was considerably lighter than at RMH, the rostered time on duty being 105 hours per week. I had to sleep at the hospital two nights a week and alternate weekends; a major improvement which was greatly appreciated as Kevin was born in March 1965.

The difference between paediatric and adult medicine was marked; in general the children recovered from their illnesses rapidly contrary to the situation at RMH where many of the patients were old with advanced chronic disease which ran a progressive downhill course despite treatment. It was particularly rewarding to watch a child desperately ill due to an acute infection respond to treatment and recover quickly. The children were a delight to treat and a bond could usually be rapidly formed with them. It was, of course, upsetting when a child died because of malignant disease or an overwhelming acute infection in which case helping the parents through the terrible situation became a priority.

Recognition of the child who was dangerously ill and whose illness was likely to progress rapidly was always in our mind. At the introductory talk we received on our first day at the hospital this point was stressed, with the warning that during the year it was likely that at least one of the RMO's would send a child home from the Emergency Department who would die within hours.

I enjoyed the year very much and did give some thought as to whether I might aim at making a career in Paediatrics. However, I had found obstetrics and gynaecology very interesting during the medical course and had always planned to gain further experience in that area.

ROYAL WOMENS HOSPITAL

I commenced work as an RMO at RWH in February 1966 immediately after completing my term at RCH.

The RWH was organised differently to the RMH and RCH.

Accommodation was provided, married couples being offered small houses in Faraday Street and Cardigan Street adjacent to the hospital and unmarried doctors were housed in the Residents Quarters within the hospital precinct. Bev and I were offered, for a nominal rent, a two-storey dwelling in Faraday Street which became our home for three years. It contained a sitting room, dining room, three bedrooms, bathroom, laundry, kitchen and an external toilet. It had minimal furniture and was sorely in need of renovation. There was further improvement in rostered working time to 82 hours per week. RMO's at RWH were on call from 8.00am to 10.00pm with one afternoon and two evenings off duty through the week and worked 48 hours on alternate weekends.

Each RMO spent one month on night duty and eleven months working in one of the five hospital units. The work load for RMO's on day duty was heavy; we attended three outpatient clinics and one operating session each week and were responsible for the care of 20 inpatients. There were two formal ward rounds with the consultant doctors of the unit each week. We had to assess and care for all patients registered to our unit who were admitted to delivery suite or who attended the Emergency Department. RMO's worked under the supervision of the unit registrar, usually a second-year trainee, who was responsible for much of our teaching, both theoretical and practical. I was allotted to the Professorial Unit, the unit head being Professor S.L. Townsend, Professor of Obstetrics and Gynaecology, University of Melbourne. The registrar of this unit was a third-year trainee who, being more experienced, was a better teacher.

One RMO was rostered to work night duty during the week but did not cover weekends. This job was very busy and stressful. The night duty RMO was responsible for bleeding any patient's relatives who volunteered to donate blood in response to a request broadcast at the end of each evening visiting hour, then returned to work from 10.00pm until 8.00am. As well as being responsible for all patients in delivery suite and any who attended the Emergency Department and all emergency situations which occurred in the wards, the night duty RMO had to group and cross match any blood required for transfusion during the night as there was no pathology technician rostered to be present in the hospital during the night.

The heavy workload ensured that RMO's rapidly developed skills in assessing patients, in resuscitation and in practical matters such as easy forcep, breech and twin deliveries. In the operating theatre they were permitted to perform most surgeries for ovarian cyst and ectopic pregnancy and a limited number of Caesarean Sections.

The outpatient clinics at RWH were very long with many patients to be seen.

Antenatal clinics were held in the morning, gynaecology clinics in the afternoon and it was common for the RMO in the antenatal clinic to be still seeing patients at 1:30pm when the gynaecology clinic commenced, which meant, of course, that the RMO did not get any lunch that day.

The gynaecology outpatient clinic I attended was followed by a formal ward round with Professor Townsend after which the RMO was rostered to attend the operating theatre to do a list of minor cases while the other members of the unit repaired to the RMO's quarters for a Friday afternoon debrief over a beer.

Theoretical teaching was obtained at regular hospital clinical meetings and at unit ward rounds. The rounds conducted by Professor Townsend were by far the best teaching sessions I attended during my entire post-graduate training; the RMO presented the patient's history, examination findings and treatment to date, then other unit members, in order of seniority, commented on management with the Professor finally summing up the situation.

~ ~ ~

I had always planned that I would spend one year of postgraduate training at each of the RMH, the RCH and the RWH and then commence General Practice, possibly with my father in Brunswick or possibly in a country town. However, having found the work at RWH so interesting, stimulating and challenging, I decided that I would endeavour to make my career in obstetrics and gynaecology. This was an emotional decision. I enjoyed the work, related well to the patients whether they be pregnant or suffering from a gynaecological condition and found great joy in delivering a baby, particularly if the delivery was complicated and difficult. I gave no thought to the negative aspects of obstetric and gynaecological practice: the irregular hours, the frequent moments of stress, the poor remuneration relative to other specialties and the concern about medico-legal matters. Accordingly I applied for, and was appointed to, a position as registrar at RWH in 1967.

The work of a registrar was an extension of the work done by RMOs with greater responsibility, a teaching role and involvement with more complicated deliveries and more demanding surgery.

Five registrars were appointed, and each spent nine months working in several of the four non-Professorial units and three months in the Pathology Department performing autopsies on babies who had been stillborn or died in the early neo-natal period and preparing and reporting on tissue removed at surgery. We also used this time to prepare a volume, *Obstetrical and Gynaecological Cases and Commentaries*, which had to satisfy the examiners of the Royal College of Obstetricians and Gynaecologists before we were permitted to sit for the examination to gain entry to the College and thereby achieve specialist recognition. This entailed providing a detailed description of fifteen obstetric and fifteen gynaecology cases we had personally managed, together with a commentary on one obstetric and one gynaecology subject which had to be of a standard suitable for publication in a medical journal.

~~~

In March 1968 I was appointed to the position of Second Assistant, Department of Obstetrics and Gynaecology, University of Melbourne. This involved spending eight months at RWH and four months working at the General Hospital, Port Moresby, Territory of Papua and New Guinea (TPNG).

At the RWH I was given a great deal of responsibility in the area of patient management and was heavily involved supervising and instructing RMOs and in providing formal lectures and clinical teaching to medical students. The latter involved taking students for ward rounds in the delivery suite, encouraging them to assist at complicated deliveries and gynaecological surgery and taking each of them through a student forcep delivery.

It has been said that the best way of learning something is to teach it and I certainly found that the heavy involvement in teaching clarified my ideas about the theory and practice of obstetrics and gynaecology; this was very important in view of the fact that I was soon to sit for the Royal College of Obstetricians and Gynaecologists entrance examination.

The work load was heavy. Second Assistants were rostered to be on duty every second weekend and for total of 110 hours a week.

GENERAL HOSPITAL, PORT MORESBY, TPNG

In July 1968, Bev and I and our three children, Kevin three years and four months, Andrew 21 months and Janine three months, travelled to Port Moresby where I was to work with the gynaecologist appointed to relieve the permanent head of the Obstetric and Gynaecology Department at the General Hospital while he took sabbatical leave. It transpired that the relieving person was unwell and unable to work; so for four months I was the sole practitioner providing obstetric and gynaecology services to the native women of Port Moresby and surrounding districts and to patients referred from other areas of TPNG. It also meant that I was permanently on duty.

The flight to Port Moresby was interesting. We took an early morning plane from Tullamarine to Sydney in order to board an international flight to Port Moresby. During the waiting time Bev took Janine to the ladies rest room to breast feed her, leaving me with the two boys, both over-excited and hyper-active, half a dozen bags to guard and five departure cards to complete. Not good at birthdays at the best of times and now under some stress I made a guess at the dates, getting two wrong – not that it seemed to matter. The air temperature at Jackson's Airport was about 25 degrees Celsius higher than it was when we left Melbourne and we had to queue in the sun to be processed by Customs and Immigration. We lost track of Andrew and found him at the custom officials table staring intently and with awe at the gentleman's huge bare black feet. We had taken a pack of playing cards, thinking they might be useful for evening entertainment, there being no television; they were a prohibited item in TPNG and we had to open a number of cases and bags in order to locate them and hand them to the custom official.

One of the senior doctors from the hospital met us and transported us and our luggage to the residence we were to occupy during our stay. He reassured us that Port Moresby was a very safe place but warned us that if we should happen to have a car accident involving an indigenous person not to get out to see if all was well but to drive straight to the police station, as the natives tended to administer summary justice.

The work in Port Moresby was fascinating, the problems encountered contrasting greatly with those seen in Melbourne. Most native women delivered their babies with minimal fuss and noise; indeed, if one cried out she was generally in big trouble. Severe anaemia was common because of malaria and an iron deficient diet; part of routine ante-natal care was administration of iron and anti-malarial therapy at each visit. Major mechanical problems precluding delivery were common and frequently had been neglected for days prior to presentation at the hospital. On a number of occasions I was involved in rescue flights in single engine Cessna aircraft to treat obstetric patients with severe problems and transport them to the hospital. Some of the rough grass air strips we used were daunting, although the pilots of the aircraft seemed to be completely unfazed and confident. TPNG is a bad place to have an engine failure as the terrain is amazingly rugged and heavily forested with no place for a safe forced landing.

We also provided medical cover for St. Therese Catholic Mission Hospital at nearby Koki village where Sister Camillus and a volunteer Australian midwife provided midwifery care to local women.

The facilities available to treat patients were far inferior to those in Melbourne; the architecture of the delivery suite was such that it was not possible to provide an anaesthetic machine to administer general anaesthesia. Caesarean section could only be performed after the patient was moved by ambulance to an operating theatre in a distant part of the hospital.

My parents took a package tour of TPNG which terminated in Port Moresby intending to spend a few days with us prior to returning to Melbourne. On the day they arrived I received a phone call telling me that my father had collapsed at Jackson's Airport, had been transported to the hospital by ambulance and been seen by a physician who had diagnosed a likely heart attack and arranged for an electrocardiogram and blood tests to be performed. When I saw him shortly after this he was pale, sweating and mentally confused with a very low blood pressure. He proceeded to vomit a large amount of blood making the diagnosis of bleeding from a chronic duodenal ulcer, which he had suffered from and had bled from on several prior occasions. I inserted an intravenous line, gave him a quick litre of fluid, arranged for a blood transfusion and for re-assessment by the physician. Fortunately the ulcer stopped bleeding and after six units of blood he was much better and ultimately able to fly home. Malaria is endemic in TPNG and all blood transfusions were accompanied by an injection of chloroquine; despite this he did get a malarial infection which caused repeated mild attacks over several years.

Port Moresby in 1966 was different to Port Moresby in the 21st Century.

Lawlessness was not an issue. We lived in a bungalow in the suburb of Boroko close to the General Hospital. The house was not fortified and there were no fences around any of the properties. We felt quite safe walking around the town and our blond haired children were often the centre of attention in the native markets, which we patronised without trepidation. The only episode of tension we witnessed was in relation to the unexpected death of a young woman in the hospital; her relatives were unhappy and made some threats to hospital staff necessitating a police presence for several days.

We had the use of an aged Volkswagon Beetle and took the opportunity to travel around Port Moresby as far as the roads would allow, a radius of about 30 kilometres from the town centre. On one such drive to Brown River on a hot day we enjoyed a picnic then took off our shoes and waded in the shallows. A passing group of natives warned us in no uncertain terms to leave the water because of the danger of crocodile attack.

~~~

On returning to Melbourne in November I resumed work at RWH and, after Christmas commenced, studying in preparation for the College entrance examination which I planned to take in April 1969. Part of the preparation involved meeting with two other candidates on a weekly basis to discuss model answers each prepared to questions which had appeared on examination papers in the last ten years. This, together with reading medical text books and journals and the clinical work and teaching I did in the hospital setting, gave a solid base of knowledge to take into the examination.

~~~

My employment at RWH ceased in March 1969 and we had to vacate the residence in Faraday Street. As we had no other home Bev and the three children moved to Nagambie where they lived with my sister Kate whilst I lived with my parents in East Ivanhoe during the week so that I could continue studying and spent the weekends with Bev and the children.

I took the College examination in April, the written examinations being held at RWH and the clinical and oral examinations at Crown Street Hospital in Sydney, where we were tested by external examiners from England. I passed the examination and was duly appointed a Member of the Royal College of Obstetricians and Gynaecologists.

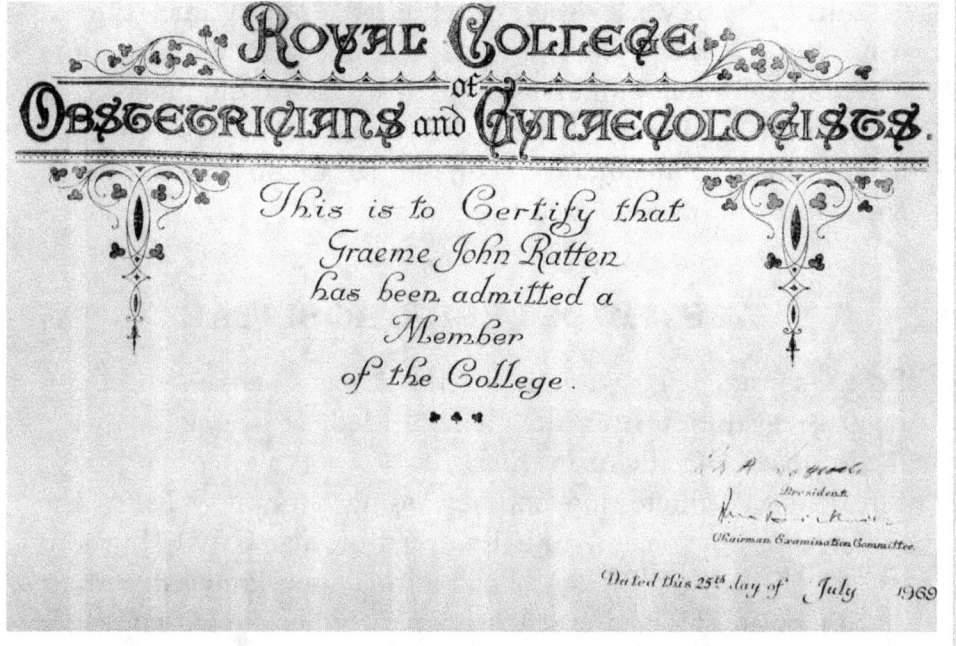

Shortly after this, Bev and I and the children, now aged four years one month, two years six months and fourteen months, boarded the liner *Australis* to travel to England where a position as registrar in obstetrics and gynaecology at West Middlesex Hospital had been arranged for me by Professor Townsend. We chose to travel by ship as the timing fitted well with the starting date for the job at West Middlesex and it was also the cheapest way to travel. It also enabled us to take much clothing and household items in trunks stored in the hold of the ship. The six week voyage was a nightmare. Due to a dock strike in Melbourne we had to travel to Sydney by train before embarking. The train, an old, superseded country model, had separate compartments capable of taking eight persons, was not air-conditioned and there was a chemical heater on the floor. It was frequently diverted onto a siding to allow regular trains to pass resulting in the journey taking fifteen hours during which time we were provided with sandwiches and bottled water. We shared the compartment with a lady who had two young children which made for a restless trip. Kevin vomited which provoked further discomfort.

During the six week voyage the children, one at a time, suffered from measles, recovered from this then repeated the procedure with chicken pox, Janine's rash appearing as we disembarked at Southampton. Bev and I spent the voyage nursing the children in the small cabin and were unable to attend the shipboard entertainment or shore excursions as a couple.

WEST MIDDLESEX HOSPITAL

Before commencing work at WMH it was necessary to obtain medial registration from the General Medical Council allowing me to practice medicine in the U.K.

I had a very interesting and rewarding time at WMH. The senior consultant of the unit I worked on, Mr C.W.F. Burnett, was a polished English gentleman with a good knowledge of art and literature. He had excellent surgical skills and his fame as a teacher was such that many candidates preparing for the College examination attended his ward rounds. He had little interest in clinical obstetrics. The senior registrar was also more interested in gynaecology and the delivery suite became my domain, an arrangement which suited me well. A great deal of gynaecological surgery was performed and I gained much experience and also learned the technique of laparoscopy, which had not been available in Melbourne. The other medical staff and the nursing staff were pleasant to work with and I enjoyed involvement in teaching student midwives, medical students, junior hospital doctors and post-graduate students.

POSTGRADUATE TRAINING

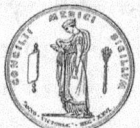

GENERAL MEDICAL COUNCIL
44 HALLAM STREET, LONDON, W.1

MEDICAL ACT, 1956

CERTIFICATE OF FULL REGISTRATION AS A MEDICAL PRACTITIONER

Registration No.: 1407251   Date of Certificate: 5 Mar 1969

I HEREBY CERTIFY that the following is a true copy of the entry in the Register relating to the fully registered medical practitioner named below :—

```
RATTEN, Graeme                        5 Mar 1969      C
        John
269 The Boulevard, Ivanhoe, Victoria, Australia
MB BS 1963 Melbourne
```

The entry in the Register reproduced above shows the name, date of full registration, address, and qualifications of the practitioner to whom it relates. If two dates are shown, the first date (distinguished by an asterisk) is that of *provisional* registration.
A letter E after the date of registration indicates that the practitioner was registered by the Registrar of the Branch Council for England and Wales. C or F indicates that the practitioner was registered as a Commonwealth or a foreign practitioner, as the case may be.

W. K. Pyke-Lees
REGISTRAR

NOTE

This certificate is given to afford immediate evidence of the registration which it attests. In due course the practitioner will be shown in the Medical Register published annually by the Council as fully registered, and reference should thereafter be made to the CURRENT Medical Register for evidence of the continued registration of the practitioner.

Spottiswoode, Ballantyne & Co. Ltd., Printers to the General Medical Council, London and Colchester.

Mr Burnett's wisdom and pragmatism was seen in his response to a rather ticklish situation we encountered; a young woman presented to the hospital with a history of mild but persistent pain for many months following life-saving abdominal surgery for a ruptured ectopic pregnancy performed at a nearby hospital. The source of the pain was obscure and eventually a laparotomy was performed and an overlooked abdominal pack removed. Justice was tempered with mercy; the pack was laundered and returned to the other hospital with an appropriate note and the patient told that she had suffered from a twisted bowel which was now pristine. This explanation undoubtedly saved the first hospital and its medical and theatre staff from considerable publicity and embarrassment and the National Health Service a significant amount of money, but did prevent a law firm from realising a windfall payment.

I was offered further employment at WMH but a junior consultant position became available at RWH, Melbourne and as this was my aim we travelled back to Melbourne, with Qantas not by ship.

~~~

Postgraduate training in obstetrics and gynaecology, as in other branches of medicine, is akin to an apprenticeship; one learns on the job while being mentored by senior experienced people. During my training I had contact with, and learned from, many knowledgeable doctors. There were four who, for various reasons, made a major contribution to my training. Professor Sir Sydney Lance Townsend taught me the importance of good organisation and of loyalty to the people with whom you work, particularly junior members of the team. Professor Norman Beischer taught me the importance of having an interest in academic medicine, in research and in preparing articles for publication. I remember Doctor Gordon Ley as the complete obstetrician, knowledgeable, caring, dextrous, unflappable – always calm in delivery suite no matter how dire the situation. Mr Vernon Hollyock taught me the importance of extreme care when operating and being meticulous with haemostasis.

Whilst the postgraduate training we received was excellent both from a theoretical and practical point of view, we received little emotional support. Excellence was expected and if our performance was unsatisfactory, we were told plainly that we needed to lift our game. When we were involved in a case with an unfortunate outcome, as occurs not infrequently in obstetrics, we were expected to support and counsel the patient and her relatives but received little, in fact usually no, support or counselling ourselves from the senior medical staff, this being received from our contemporaries usually over a beer at the end of the day. This led to a degree of 'emotional toughening' which probably resulted in an improved ability to perform well under situations of extreme stress; important as the person in charge of a fraught situation in the delivery suite or operating theatre needs to remain calm and lead the team conducting the resuscitation and correction of the problem.

CHANGES IN POSTGRADUATE TRAINING

Postgraduate training in the 21st Century differs greatly from training in the 1960s. Trainees no longer work such challenging hours and therefore twice as many are needed to provide clinical care of hospital patients, thus diluting their experience.

There has been a swing away from manipulative obstetrics, largely driven by fear of medical litigation and many twins and babies in breech presentation or requiring midforcep delivery are now treated by caesarean section.

Many gynaecological conditions previously treated by major surgery are now amenable to treatment with hormone preparations or by highly specialised minimal invasive surgery techniques not available to the general trainee.

These factors have led to a dilution of experience and the training program is now much longer. I received my postgraduate training over six and a half years of which four and a half were devoted to obstetrics and gynaecology. Nowadays most trainees spend three years gaining general experience before being accepted into an obstetric and gynaecology training program, which involves a minimum of six years often with a further two years of sub-specialty training; thus a minimum of eleven years postgraduate training. Even so, their experience and skills in manipulative obstetric delivery and gynaecological surgery is inferior to that obtained by trainees in the 1960's.

CHANGE IN COLLEGE STRUCTURE

In 1979, an Australian College of Obstetricians and Gynaecologists was formed and all Australian Members and Fellows of the Royal College were admitted as Foundation Fellows (FAGO).

The Australian College of Obstetricians & Gynaecologists

This is to certify that

Graeme John Ratten

has been admitted a
FOUNDATION FELLOW
of the College

Dated this 31st. day of August, 1979.

PRESIDENT:

HONORARY SECRETARY:

In 1982, by virtue of the passage of time, I was offered the opportunity to upscale from Member of the Royal College of Obstetricians and Gynaecologists (MRCOG) to Fellow (FRCOG).

ROYAL COLLEGE of OBSTETRICIANS and GYNAECOLOGISTS

This is to Certify that

GRAEME JOHN RATTEN

has been admitted a Fellow
of the College

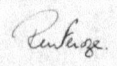 President

Dated this 2nd day of June 19 82

In subsequent years the Australian College received Royal assent and became the Royal Australian College of Obstetricians and Gynaecologists (RACOG). Amalgamation with the New Zealand College occurred and I was appointed a Fellow of the Royal Australian and New Zealand College of Obstetricians and Gynaecologists. (FRANZOG).

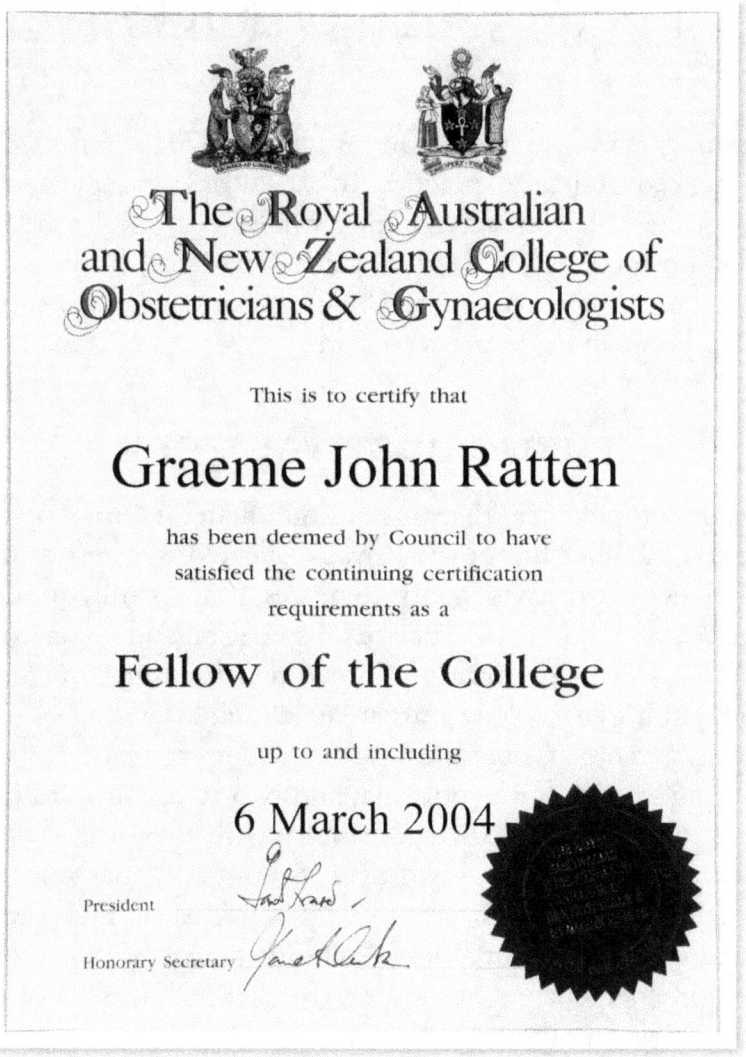

A CAREER IN OBSTETRICS AND GYNAECOLOGY

Returning from England in August 1970, I immediately commenced full-time practice in obstetrics and gynaecology. There were three aspects to this career – clinical work with public hospital patients, with private patients, and academic and teaching responsibilities. There was, of course, considerable overlap between these facets of work.

PUBLIC HOSPITAL WORK

Having completed a rigorous postgraduate training program, achieved membership of the Royal College of Obstetricians and Gynaecologists and with good references, I successfully applied for a position of Honorary Associate Obstetrician and Gynaecologist at RWH. This involved caring for women attending an antenatal clinic and a gynaecology outpatient clinic, attending one four-hour gynaecology operating session, one two-hour obstetric operating session and two formal and two informal ward rounds each week. I also shared responsibility with two other honorary consultant doctors for providing 168 hours of emergency cover per week. These duties generated a workload which required attendance at RWH for at least 20 hours per week and an on-call roster for emergency situations for a further 56 hours per week. As an honorary appointee no salary or travelling allowance was paid to compensate for this work. The honorary appointment however carried the right to admit private patients to the hospital, to care for them in the hospital delivery suites and operating theatres, to maintain knowledge and expertise by attending clinical meetings held at the hospital and to have access to the wisdom and experience of senior staff members when dealing with difficult clinical situations.

As well as being directly involved in the care of patients in the outpatient clinics, wards, operating theatres and delivery suites, Honorary Consultant Obstetricians and Gynaecologists had a major role in the theoretical teaching and practical instruction of RMOs and in direct supervision of their work in complicated situations and in teaching of medical students.

I held the position of Honorary Associate Obstetrician and Gynaecologist for four years and was then appointed to the position of Honorary Obstetrician. This elevation in status absolved me from responsibility for public gynaecology patients but I had greater responsibility for public obstetric patients.

In 1976 staffing of public hospitals by honorary consultants ceased and I became a consultant obstetrician and was paid a salary for sessional work I performed and a call-back allowance for emergency attendances out-of-hours.

I continued to care for public obstetric patients at RWH until I retired from the hospital in 1996.

Like all members of the Department of Obstetrics, I spent one year as Chair of the department. A meeting was held each month at which matters affecting the practice of obstetrics at the hospital were discussed and, if necessary, recommendations forwarded to the senior medical staff for further consideration. If deemed necessary, the matter could then be referred to the Hospital Committee of Management for further discussion.

I also spent several years as secretary of the senior medical staff which met at monthly intervals and represented the Department of Obstetrics on the Hospital Building Committee.

In 1971 I was invited to take up a position of First Assistant (part-time) in the University Department of Obstetrics and Gynaecology at the Mercy Maternity Hospital (later called the Mercy Hospital for Women). This was a salaried position and entailed involvement in teaching medical students and in research work. It carried with it an appointment as Honorary Associate Obstetrician and Gynaecologist at MMH which involved weekly attendance at an antenatal clinic and responsibility for out-of-hours management of obstetric and gynaecology emergencies.

In 1976, with the dismantling of the honorary consultant system, the position was re-named Associate Obstetrician and Gynaecologist and carried a salary of one session per week and payment for on-call attendance out-of-hours.

I held these appointments of First Assistant (part-time) and Associate Obstetrician and Gynaecologist at MMH until 1984 and continued to attend the weekly antenatal clinic until retirement in 2009.

CARE FOR PRIVATE PATIENTS

On my return to Melbourne, Mr Vernon Hollyock, Senior Gynaecologist at RWH, offered me use of his consulting rooms on the 9th floor of 20 Collins Street, Melbourne and it was from here that I conducted my obstetric and gynaecology private practice for the next 22 years. Vern was a friend of my father and had, for a time, worked in his general practice and had known me since I was aged 10 years. Like many senior gynaecologists he was in the process of ceasing obstetric practice and was happy for me to care for any of his patients who became pregnant. In return I provided cover for his practice on alternate weekends, and we frequently assisted each other with surgical cases. As Vern approached retirement his practice decreased in size and he needed less time in the consulting rooms which was balanced by my need for more time as my practice increased in size.

As a junior specialist many senior gynaecologists asked me to provide locum cover for their private practice at weekends and when they took holidays and to assist them with surgical cases. I was, of course, delighted to provide this service until after a couple of years my own practice was large enough to support me financially and did not allow time to provide these services to others.

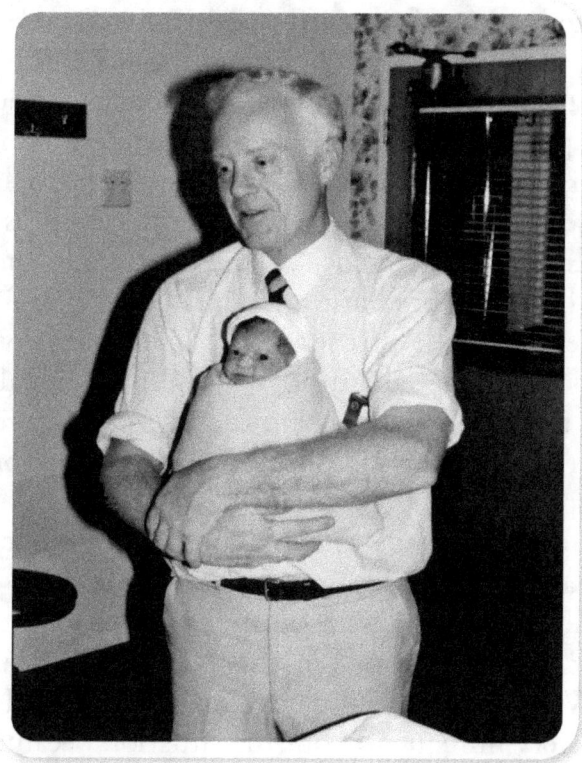

In the early 1970s many general practitioners delivered babies in small local hospitals and much of my work in the early years involved attending such hospitals to perform rescue forcep deliveries and Caesarean Sections when the process of labour had gone awry. This work was challenging and disruptive as the emergencies occurred without warning at any time of day or night, but I found it extremely interesting and rewarding. There is no better emotion than the one which occurs after safely delivering a baby from a hazardous situation. This work also generated much routine work as the doctors whose patient I had delivered frequently referred other patients for opinion and management. Indeed, it was one such episode which led to a relationship with the doctors of Livingstone Street Clinic, Ivanhoe General Practice, whereby I saw many of their obstetric patients in late pregnancy and managed their labour and delivery and also cared for their patients with gynaecological conditions.

The introduction of expensive and sophisticated technology to monitor the wellbeing of the baby during labour is one of the reasons that small suburban hospitals no longer provide birthing facilities. Equally as important is the fact that metropolitan general practitioners, who provided most of the care in such hospitals, have decided that the care of women in labour is so poorly remunerated and leads to such a large increase in their medical indemnity insurance premiums that it is not economically viable to continue to provide this service. While general practitioners still provide care for labouring women in regional hospitals, women in metropolitan areas are forced to seek care in public hospitals or with private obstetricians in large city or suburban private hospitals.

Two of the issues gynaecologists must face are termination of early pregnancy and sterilization. The MHW and the RWH have diametrically opposed views regarding these procedures. Neither operation can be performed at the MHW, a Roman Catholic hospital. When I commenced my training at RWH both were performed very infrequently but the situation became relaxed as the years passed and social attitudes and the law changed.

My practice was to readily perform sterilization but to only terminate early pregnancies if the mother suffered from a condition that made it life threatening for her to be pregnant, or if the foetus had a major abnormality.

As my private practice increased in volume, I was able to centralise it, both obstetrics and gynaecology, to RWH and MHW thereby ensuring that all clinical work, both public and private, was restricted to those two hospitals.

ACADEMIC AND TEACHING RESPONSIBILITY

Teaching has played an important role in my career. I have been involved in providing formal lectures to midwifery and undergraduate and postgraduate medical students and informal teaching by way of inpatient ward rounds, outpatient clinics and assessment of women in delivery suite.

Both RWH and MMH are teaching hospitals for midwifery and medical students, and students attended every delivery in which I was involved, whether the patient was public or private; a student scrubbed up to assist with or to perform the delivery under close supervision. Interestingly no private patient ever complained about student involvement in her delivery.

As an examiner I have been involved in assessment of undergraduate medical students and of postgraduate students taking the examination for the Diploma or Membership of the Royal Australian and New Zealand College of Obstetricians and Gynaecologists. Since 1996 I have been a senior examiner for the Australian Medical Council assessing overseas trained doctors for suitability to obtain Australian Registration.

I was fortunate to be associated with University Departments thereby being involved in research work and the production of original articles suitable for publication in medical journals. I owe a debt of gratitude to Professor Norman Beischer whose energy and intellectual drive stimulated me in this area. The 31 original articles I have had published in refereed journals are tabulated at the end of this chapter (Table 1).

I served for 10 years as an Associate Editor of the Australian and New Zealand Journal of Obstetrics and Gynaecology.

~~~

My time was spent approximately 50/50 with private patients/public hospital patients and administration. My private practice was approximately 50/50 obstetrics and gynaecology.

It is of interest to document the amount of clinical work performed during the 22 years of full-time clinical work and the figures are tabled at the end of the chapter (Table 2). The figures for private patients are accurate, those for public hospital work are approximations. They include deliveries and surgical procedures performed during my postgraduate training and the patients I operated on as a consultant. No count has been kept of the number of curettes or repairs of episiotomy I performed but each would have numbered several thousand.

This clinical work-load generated many attendances by patients to the consulting rooms and led to problems with time management. I have frequently heard patients complain that consultations with their doctor were rushed; in an attempt to ameliorate this I made it a habit to try and remember to ask each patient at every visit if they had any questions they wanted to ask. Consulting room sessions can be a nightmare for a busy obstetrician as one will invariably be frequently called to attend the delivery suite. I was fortunate to have receptionists with the ability to cope with patients unhappy about the delay and to be prepared to work past their usual finishing time.

~~~

In 1992 after 22 years of full-time private and public clinical practice I made the decision that it was time to ease my workload. During those years I was perpetually on call apart from four weeks holiday each year and 36 hours every second weekend which were usually spent at Nagambie and occasional evenings during which times Doctor Lou Butterfield covered my practice. In return I looked after Lou's patients on alternate weekends and when he took annual leave. I carried a paging device all the time and Bev and I travelled to church and to all social activities in separate cars because of the likelihood of emergency calls. I was called to the delivery suite during the night twice a week on average and received a telephone call for advice on another two occasions. These telephone calls at night, taken during a period of deep sleep, were sometimes the source of some confusion. Bev occasionally had to intervene to ensure that I had not fallen back to sleep nor was talking absolute nonsense to the hospital nurse or patient who had rung. Interruptions to sleep was dealt with by developing the ability to catnap at other times, a talent that I retain to this day. I do recall driving home on one occasion at 3.00am after attending delivery suite at RWH and being delayed at the Australian Paper Mill in Heidelberg Road, Fairfield by a train which was used to move material from the factory to the nearby suburban rail network. I waited patiently and fell asleep to be awakened by the insistent sounding of the car horn from the vehicle behind me.

By 1992 three of our children were married and financially independent and only Nicola, who was still at University, remained at home; this meant that I could afford to lessen my workload.

The Deputy Medical Superintendent at RWH resigned and the hospital decided to replace him with a Clinical Services Manager, a position which was 70/30 administration/public hospital clinical work. Having applied for and being appointed to this position I was able to cease all private practice, this being the most demanding work in terms of out-of-hours calls. The position of Clinical Services Manager involved, as the name suggests, ensuring that clinical services, medical and ancillary were delivered as efficiently and as effectively as possible. To this end I organised the rosters for the junior medical staff, arranged a lecture program for them and counselled them if their performance was sub-standard.

I worked with the Patient Representative who was the first port of call for patients who were unhappy with the treatment they had received, often meeting with them to explain the clinical situation they had encountered. I responded to enquiries from legal practitioners retained by disgruntled patients and worked with the lawyers retained by the hospital to represent it and on occasion attended court as the hospital's legal representative.

A useful innovation, developed with input from the patient representative, was an occasional newsletter circulated widely within the hospital which highlighted various situations in which the performance of hospital staff, both medical and nursing, was either sub-standard or inappropriate. Names of patients and of the staff involved were, of course, carefully concealed. As one would expect the problems frequently had their genesis in careless, inaccurate or thoughtless communication and the newsletter was helpful in improving the performance of hospital staff.

I continued to work with one of the hospital's obstetric units providing care to antenatal, labouring and postnatal women.

This mix of administration and clinical work was interesting and stimulating. The difference made to our life-style was enormous. With limited out-of-hours duty Bev and I could now travel to social gatherings in one car.

I continued as Clinical Services Manager for four years until 1996 when the RWH reorganised its administration service. I decided that it was time to take another step towards total retirement. Although I continued to attend a weekly antenatal clinic at Mercy Hospital for Women until 2009, I no longer had responsibility for inpatient care and had no more calls to the delivery suite.

~~~

There have been major changes in the practice of obstetrics and gynaecology in the 52 years since I commenced postgraduate training as there has been in all branches of medicine. As in other specialties the most obvious changes have been in the development and availability of new, more effective drugs and in technological advances which enhance diagnostic capabilities and enable therapy to be administered more safely, effectively, and efficiently.

In gynaecology, development of drugs to treat infertility and of hormone preparations which can be used to treat various disorders of menstruation are obvious changes. Similarly, more effective chemotherapeutic agents have revolutionised the management of gynaecological cancers. Minimally invasive surgical techniques allow treatment of many conditions to be performed with the patient requiring much less time in hospital and returning to normal activities more rapidly.

Changes in obstetric practice are even more pronounced. Prenatal counselling is now recommended so that the possible presence of inherited disease can be explored and, if necessary, appropriate genetic testing arranged. It is recommended that folic acid be taken prior to conception and during the first trimester to minimise the risk of central nervous system deformities. Antenatal testing of the foetus for genetic abnormalities such as Down Syndrome are readily available. Ultrasound scans have given obstetricians the ability to diagnose many foetal abnormalities and to assess foetal growth and wellbeing and even correct some abnormalities while the baby is still in utero. Ready availability of more effective methods of alleviating pain have resulted in labour being much less of an ordeal than in former years.

There has been a marked increase in the incidence of Caesarean delivery. The Caesarean Section rate in public hospitals was 4% when I commenced my training and is now 30% and even higher in private patients. Some of the increase is due to a reluctance to undertake difficult vaginal deliveries resulting in a decrease in the number of forcep deliveries. Twin pregnancies and babies presenting by the breech are now commonly delivered by Caesarean Section. Importantly a more humane attitude has led to the abandonment of long difficult labours.

When I commenced practice in 1970, and for most of my career in obstetrics and gynaecology, services were provided in public hospitals or by specialists most of whom were in solo private practice with loose informal arrangements with other practitioners who provided cover when they were not available. Appropriately, there had been change in this area; many obstetricians and gynaecologists now work in group practices so they can enjoy regular time off duty.

TABLE 1: PUBLICATIONS

Ratten G.J.	*Spontaneous Haematoma of the Umbilical Cord*, Aust. N.Z.J. Obstet. Gynae.,9:125 (1969)
Ratten G.J., Booth P.B	*Postpartum haemorrhage due to constitutional hypofibrinogenaemia*, Med. J. Aust., 2:1210 (1969)
Ratten G.J.	*The management of missed abortion*, Aust. N.Z.J. Obstet. Gynae. 10:115 (1970)
Ratten G.J.	*Removal of an intraperitoneal intrauterine device under laparoscopic control*, Med. J. Aust. 2:1977 (1971)

Ratten G.J., Beischer N.A.	*The significance of anaemia in an obstetric population in Australia*, J. Obstet. Gynae. Brit. Cwlth., 3:79 (1972)
Ratten G.J.	*Resumption of ovulation after incomplete abortion*, Aust. N.Z.J. Obstet. Gynae. 12:217 (1972)
Ratten G.J., Beischer N.A., Fortune D.W.	*Obstetric complications when the fetus has Potter's Syndrome: Part 1. Clinical considerations*, Amer. J. Obstet. Gynae. 115:890 (1973)
Beischer N.A. Ratten G.J., Fortune D.W., Macafee J.	*Obstetric complications when the fetus has Potter' Syndrome: Part 2. Fetoplacental function*, Amer. J. Obstet. Gynae. 116:62 (1973)
Ratten G.J., Beischer N.A.	*The effect of maternal anaemia on the fetoplacental unit*, Ob/Gyn. Digest (1974)
Ratten G.J., Kenny J.M., Targett C.S., Beischer N.A.	*The effect of maternal socio-economic status on fetal and placental weight at birth*, Aust. N.Z.J. Obstet. Gynae 14:149 (1974)
Ratten G.J., Targett C.S., Drew J.H., Beischer N.A.	*The effect of fetal and placental weight at birth on weight during early childhood*, Med. J. Aust., 2:735 (1975)
Paull J.D., Ratten G. J.	*Ergometrine and third stage blood loss*, Med J. Aust., 1:178 (1977)
Targett C.S., Ratten G.J., Abell D.A., Beischer N.A.	*The influence of smoking on intrauterine fetal growth and on maternal oestriol excretion*, Aust. N.Z.J. Obstet. Gynae. 17:126 (1977)
Ratten G.J., Beischer N.A.	*The influence of maternal weight loss on the outcome of pregnancy*, Aust. N.Z.J. Obstet. Gynae. 17:121 (1977)

Ratten G.J.	*The use of drugs in pregnancy and labour*, Australian Family Physician 9:118 (1978)
Wein P.E., Ratten G.J.	*Acute polyhydramnios – A complication of monozygous twin pregnancy*, Brit. J. Obstet. Gynae. 86:849 (1979)
Ratten G.J., Beischer N.A.	*The effect of termination of pregnancy on maturity of subsequent pregnancy*, Med. J. Aust. 1:479 (1979)
Ratten G.J.	*Practical obstetric procedures*, Patient Management 75 (1980
Ratten G.J.	*"Prolonged pregnancy" after oral contraceptive*, Therapy Med. J. Aust. 1:641 (1981)
Ratten G.J.	*Aetiology of delivery during the second trimester and performance in subsequent pregnancies*, Med J. Aust. 2:654 (1981)
Ratten G.J.	*Cervical pregnancy treated by ligation of the descending branch of the uterine arteries*, Brit. J. Obstet. Gynae. 90:367 (1983)
Ashton P., Beischer N.A., Cullen J., Ratten G.J.	*Return to theatre – Experience at the Mercy Maternity Hospital 1971-1982*, Aust. N.Z.J. Obstet. Gynae. 25:159 (1985)
Ratten G.J.	*Changes in obstetric practice in our time*, Aust. N.Z.J. Obstet. Gynae. 25:241 (1985)
Ratten G.J.	*How to manage postpartum bleeding*, Hospital Therapeutics Oct. 1987
Ratten G.J.	*Amniotic fluid embolism-two case reports and a review of maternal deaths from this cause in Australia*, Aust. N.Z. J. Obstet. Gynae. 28:33 (1988)

Wein P., Robertson B., Ratten G.J.	*Cardiorespiratory collapse and pulmonary oedema due to intravascular absorption of Prostaglandin F2 administered extra-amniotically for midtrimester termination of pregnancy*, Aust. N.Z.J. Obstet. Gynae. 29:261 (1989
Ratten G.J., McDonald L.	*Organisation and early results of a shared ante-natal program*, Aust. N.Z.J. Obstet. Gynae. 32:296 (1992)
Beischer N.A., Desmedt E., Ratten G.J., Sheedy M.,	*The significance of recurrent polyhydramnios* Aust. N.Z.J. Obstet. Gynae. 33:25 (1993)
Ratten G.J.	*Career paths of obstetricians and gynaecologists trained at the Royal Womens Hospital, Melbourne*, Aust. N.Z.J. Obstet. Gynae. 37:74 (1997)
Ratten G.J.	*Medicolegal matters involving a major obstetric and gynaecological teaching hospital*, Aust. N.Z.J. Obstet. Gynae. 37:192 (1997)
Ratten G.J.	*Enjoying retirement (Advice from the Antipodes)* Newsletter of the Retired Fellows and Members Society. RCOG April 2017

TABLE 2: CLINICAL WORK PERFORMED

PRIVATE PATIENTS

OBSTETRICS	NUMBER
Women delivered	6013
Babies born	6083
Twins	66 pairs
Twin deliveries – vaginal	53
Twin deliveries – Caesarean	13
Triplets	2 Sets
Breech deliveries	203
Caesarean Sections	691
Infant circumcisions	928

GYNAECOLOGY	NUMBER
Hysterectomy	431
Ovarian cyst	42
Ectopic pregnancy	26
Sterilization	890
Surgery for prolapse	156

PUBLIC PATIENTS

OBSTETRICS

Women delivered	approximately 4,000

GYNAECOLOGY

Major cases	approximately 210

SOME CLINICAL PROBLEMS

One of the attractions of obstetrics and gynaecology as a career is that most patients are young and healthy. Most pregnant women are happy, excited, and looking forward to becoming a mother. The obstetrician has the opportunity to develop good rapport with the patient and to share the joy following a successful pregnancy and delivery. It is important, however, to note that not all pregnancies are successful, and that appropriate management of these situations is extremely important. In similar vein many, but certainly not all, gynaecological conditions are amenable to treatment.

Threatened miscarriage, vaginal bleeding in early pregnancy, complicates one in four pregnancies; in half of these the bleeding ceases and the pregnancy continues while in half the bleeding continues and the pregnancy is lost. Many patients are devastated by this complication and all require appropriate counselling which emphasizes that miscarriage is common and has not been caused by any of the patient's actions. It should be stressed that the pregnancy resulted from the fusion of two cells, ovum and spermatozoa, which then developed into a baby and placenta; an extremely complicated process with the opportunity for something to go amiss resulting in miscarriage. Losing a pregnancy in this way does not increase the risk of miscarriage occurring in a subsequent pregnancy; it will still be one chance in six.

Stillbirth, delivery of a potentially viable baby which has died in utero occurs one in 150 pregnancies. There are many possible causes: acute infections and chronic disease processes affecting the mother, pregnancy complications such as bleeding and high blood pressure, foetal abnormalities and malfunction of the placenta. If a cause is found it is likely that appropriate treatment may enable a subsequent pregnancy to be successful. In many cases no cause is apparent and the likelihood of the next pregnancy being successful is high. The patient who suffers a stillbirth and her partner require support in several areas: information regarding the possible cause of the mishap, prognosis for the future and advice about how to cope with return to everyday life. Close supervision and much support will be needed during a future pregnancy.

Foetal abnormality which will require therapy or is uncorrectable occurs in 2% of all babies delivered. The incidence is lower now than it was 50 years ago because prenatal diagnosis has led to termination of many pregnancies in which the foetus has a chromosome abnormality or a major central nervous system defect. Among the commonest abnormalities requiring correction are heart defects, congenital dislocation of the hip, hypospadias and cleft lip/palate. The mother of children suffering such complications require a great deal of support from medical and nursing staff. I found that putting them in contact with women who had been delivered of a child with a similar problem was very helpful.

Death of a mother during pregnancy, whilst in labour, or shortly after delivery is uncommon, one in 15,000 pregnancies. I have been personally involved with only one such case, a patient undergoing elective Caesarean Section for a major degree of placenta praevia who died on the operating table from amniotic fluid embolism, a very rare, unpredictable and unavoidable condition. Informing and supporting the partner is, of course, the main issue here and requires appropriate utilisation of the resources of the hospital and its staff.

~ ~ ~

During a busy career in clinical medicine, practitioners meet and have to deal with many unusual problems. Obstetricians and gynaecologists certainly get their share of such cases and it may be of interest to consider a few that I have encountered.

Miss A, an unmarried woman, had been delivered of a child in Lebanon. The child had been adopted by her older sister and Miss A had migrated to Australia to begin a new life. She had fallen in love with a Lebanese man. They planned to marry in six months and it was important that she appear to be a virgin on her wedding night. The problem was compounded by the fact that the child had weighed four kilograms at birth and she had not required any sutures. The simple answer was to perform a vaginal repair operation enthusiastically in order to narrow the vaginal entrance to an appropriate circumference.

Mrs B, a student midwife pregnant for the first time, had an uneventful antenatal course until her husband, an intern at a Melbourne hospital, rang me at 10.00pm to say that she had been suffering nausea and headache for three days. He had diagnosed migraine and treated her accordingly with little response and she had now become blind. When I saw her at 10:30pm her blood pressure was 210/120, her urine contained protein, and the diagnosis of severe pre-eclampsia was obvious. She was in early labour, this having been masked by the drugs given for her 'migraine', and was totally blind. She required urgent treatment with drugs to control her blood pressure and to minimize the risk of an eclamptic fit. This was done and she was delivered normally of a healthy infant six hours later. Her visual loss, in retrospect due to vascular spasm caused by the severe pre-eclampsia, gradually disappeared during the following week.

Miss C, a 17-year-old from Broadmeadows, attended for a postnatal check six weeks after a normal delivery. Her pregnancy and labour had been uncomplicated and the main reason for her attendance was to arrange appropriate contraception. I checked the baby which was healthy and well-nourished and enquired as to whether it was breast fed. 'No, it was bottle fed'. 'What are you giving it?' 'Big M', she replied, 'he likes the chocolate one'. This is not ideal for a six week old child and, although he was obviously thriving, review by a hospital paediatrician was arranged so that, hopefully, a more appropriate formula could be substituted for Big M.

Miss D, a 16-year-old who had not received any antenatal care, presented to the hospital in well-established labour. We were able to measure her blood pressure and examine her abdomen but any attempt to perform a vaginal examination was met with extreme resistance and loud screams. An attempt to administer an epidural anaesthetic in the hope that a proper examination could be made was unsuccessful due to her inability to stay still. Finally, after she had been in labour for 15 hours, a light general anaesthetic was given; vaginal examination showed the cervix to be three-quarters dilated. The membranes were ruptured, and labour allowed to continue for a further six hours. Another general anaesthetic was given; the cervix was now fully dilated, and delivery was effected with forceps.

Mrs E, aged 19 years, suffered from severe anaemia due to frequent heavy menstrual periods. Her uterus was greatly enlarged and distorted by numerous fibroids, tumours consisting of muscle tissue which are common in older women but rare in women of this age. Following blood transfusion curettage was performed but the heavy periods continued, and severe anaemia recurred. Hormone therapy was not helpful so abdominal surgery was performed with many of the fibroids being removed. Unfortunately, it was impossible to remove all fibroids without compromising her uterus. It was suggested that she attempt to conceive. Fibroids are often associated with infertility, but she became pregnant after two heavy periods. The pregnancy continued normally until 38 weeks' gestation when the baby was noted to be lying in an abnormal position due to distortion of the uterus by the remaining fibroids. Caesarean Section was performed, and she was delivered of a healthy child. It was obvious that her menses would continue to be heavy so it was suggested that she should breast feed the baby for 12 months then conceive a second child. This she did and was delivered by Caesarean Section and a hysterectomy was performed at the age of 23 years.

Mrs F, a lapsed Roman Catholic, was married to a man of strict Jewish faith who insisted that their child be circumcised according to Jewish tradition. Mrs F agreed but refused to allow a Rabbi to perform the procedure. There was much argument, which was finally resolved when they requested that I act as a surrogate Rabbi – I performed the circumcision before a crowd of male onlookers while the husband read aloud from the Torah.

Mrs G presented to hospital suffering a miscarriage at 11 weeks' gestation. It was necessary for her to have a curette to ensure that no placental tissue remained in the uterus. Dental hygiene had been neglected and she had eight or ten long discoloured teeth placed randomly towards the front of her jaws. The anaesthetist managed to knock one of these and loosen it; at the end of the procedure, we straightened it and pushed it back into its socket.

Dental problems are common in public hospital patients and sufferers are generally referred to the outpatient clinic at the nearby dental hospital. On this occasion we elected to invite the hospital consulting dentist to attend and review the patient. He sat on the edge of the bed, looked at her teeth, removed the loose one with his fingers, tossed it in the bin and suggested she ring his secretary for an appointment at which time he would extract the remaining teeth and arrange for dentures to be made. After he had gone, I rescued the tooth from the rubbish bin and sent it through the internal mail system with an appropriate note to the anaesthetist as a trophy from the procedure. He, entering the spirit of the occasion, had the hospital carpenter mount it on a piece of polished red gum and hung it on the wall of his office.

On arriving in the car park of RWH one morning I noted a group of nurses surrounding a woman who was lying on the ground struggling violently and screaming loudly. She was a Greek lady who had delivered her baby after getting out of the car which had transported her to hospital and the baby was lying inside the leg of the voluminous pyjamas she was wearing. The nurses were trying to remove the pyjama pants and she was resisting strongly. The answer was to take a pair of scissors from one of the nurses and cut open the leg of the pyjamas thereby freeing the baby and allowing her to maintain her dignity.

Emotions can run high in difficult obstetric cases particularly if the outcome is bad. I arrived at RWH one Saturday morning to do a round of delivery suite to find that the husband of a woman whose baby had been stillborn during the night wandering around the hospital with a .22 rifle looking for the RMO who had been on duty. He was not aggressive to anyone else, so I engaged him in conversation to restrict his movement while the nursing staff rang the police to come and remove him. Explanation of the circumstances surrounding the stillbirth went someway to calming the situation.

Unreasonable or unattainable expectations can also be the source of anxiety and tension.

When Mrs H attended the public antenatal clinic at RWH for her initial visit in her first pregnancy her husband stated that he did not want anyone to touch what he euphemistically called her 'parts'. My response was to point out that this plan might cause considerable difficulty with delivery of the baby. The couple attended the clinic regularly and insisted that I see them at each visit. There was much discussion about the problem, and it was eventually agreed that a female doctor or midwife could touch her 'parts' as long as there was no male person in the room. The problem became more complicated when we found that it was a twin pregnancy as vaginal delivery might require the presence of a senior doctor most of whom were male. Mr H became rather aggressive about the matter and declared that if a male person did 'interfere' with his wife he would place, and detonate, a bomb within the hospital precinct. He also started telephoning me at home to reinforce his demands.

Mr H refused the offer of consultation with other medical staff including the hospital psychiatrist, the latter expressing the opinion that his paranoia was such that he could well carry out the threats he made but that involvement of the police or involuntary mental health care would not be helpful and might indeed inflame the situation. I felt nervous enough to suggest to the Director of Medical Services that the hospital take a short-term insurance policy on my life until Mrs H was safely delivered.

Eventually Mrs H's twins were delivered by Caesarean Section without her 'parts' being violated. Postnatal follow-up and counselling were refused. Sadly, we heard several years later that Mr H had killed his wife during a violent disagreement.

JOURNEY IN FARMING

My interest in farming was kindled at the age of 11 years when my father purchased a property at Nagambie. Initially covering 640 acres (one square mile) it was enlarged over the next 20 years by acquisition of adjacent paddocks as they became available; I joined with my father in the purchase of some of these. Eventually the property covered 1,200 acres.

The original manager Campbell O'Day, and his wife Mary, lived in the three bedroom and sleep-out iron roofed weatherboard dwelling and our family stayed in the home at weekends and holiday times. Typical of farmhouses in the area at that time there was no electricity and we relied on candles, Tilley lanterns and a kerosene refrigerator; there were no fans or cooling devices available nor heating apart from wood fires. The toilet was located 50 metres from the house and emptying the four-gallon drum used as a receptacle was not a favoured task. Water for the house was collected from the roof into two four-thousand-gallon tanks and had to be used sparingly; water for the garden was pumped from a nearby dam. The kitchen boasted a wood-fired stove and water for the bath was warmed by a chip heater. The telephone, Nagambie 110, shared a party-line with several adjacent properties; making a call involved cranking a handle on the telephone assembly to raise the local exchange which was staffed 24 hours a day and asking for the number desired; the telephonist could plug you directly into a local number but calls to Melbourne had to be routed through trunk lines and often entailed a significant wait, particularly in the evenings or on public holidays. One was allotted three minutes after which time the telephonist would break into the conversation to ask if you wished to extend for a further three minutes.

In succeeding years changes were made to improve living conditions. A diesel powered 32-volt electrical system was installed and eventually the State Electricity Commission brought mains power to the area. A toilet was installed in the house served by a septic system and the original out-house decommissioned. A more modern Agar wood stove was installed which also provided hot water which was plumbed to the kitchen sink, bathroom, and laundry.

As Cam and Mary's family increased the accommodation in the farmhouse became crowded and a house was purchased in Nagambie. Goulburn House was an original homestead built in 1890 by a stock and station agent. A large slate-roofed double brick dwelling with three bedrooms, two large reception rooms and a tacky weatherboard add-on containing bathroom, laundry, sleep-out and verandah, it was in need of modernisation and decoration and was set on a two-and-a-half-acre block. This enabled the family to live more comfortably and to entertain guests, something which had not previously been possible.

Five years after purchase of the farm, in 1955, Cam O'Day, a returned soldier, was offered a soldier settlement block and Harold Loughnane with wife Rhonda became manager of the property and remained so until it was sold 40 years later.

Rhonda and Harold became close friends and the children, Bev and I had many happy times with them, both at Nagambie, in Melbourne and at various holiday venues. One memorable holiday was a package tour with AAT Kings to the Red Centre taken by a group of eleven, Rhonda and Harold, two other Nagambie friends, my mother and the six of our family.

~~~

I became very involved with the farm and spent many weekends and most school holidays working as a labourer with the manager. I learned to drive the farm utility at the age of 11 years and to shoot with a rifle and shotgun and developed the skills one needs on a mixed farm: to milk a cow, to repair damaged post and wire fences and to erect new ones, to crutch sheep and trim their feet, to mark lambs and calves, to drive a tractor with plough, harrows or seeder attached and to kill, skin and butcher a sheep. I particularly enjoyed shearing time when, as a roustabout, I was responsible for helping muster and yard the sheep, fill the shearer's pens, pick up the shorn fleece and throw it on the classing table, sweep the shearing floor before the shearer brought in the next sheep, then press the classed wool into bales. Less attractive was the task of sewing bags containing harvested grain; prior to the bulk handling currently used, grain was emptied from the harvester into bags which stood in the paddock and had to be topped up then closed with a running stitch prior to being lifted onto a trailer. Bags of oats weighing 120 pounds (55 kilograms) were then taken to a shed and stacked while bags of wheat weighing 180 pounds (82 kilograms) were transported to the silo at the Nagambie railway yards.

I greatly enjoyed this aspect of life and felt that, to some extent, I was repaying my father for keeping me as I pursued my full-time secondary and tertiary education which allowed little time for part-time paid work.

My father died following a cerebral vascular episode in 1975 and I took over the running of the Nagambie property and ultimately purchased it from his estate.

There was no irrigation and stocking rates varied according to the seasons. On average we ran 1,200 – 1,500 first cross ewes (progeny of a Merino ewe and a Border Leicester ram) which cut fairly coarse wool and joined them with Southdown, Border Leicester or Perendale rams to produce fat lambs. We ran 40-80 beef cattle, mainly Hereford or Angus which were joined with a Red Pole or Charalais bull to produce vealers which were sold at six to eight months of age. In good years we would cut 50-100 acres of grass hay to store in the hayshed for use in winter and grow 100 acres of wheat or oats.

Harold and I frequently went spotlight shooting for rabbits and foxes often taking the children with us. We were usually successful and on one occasion obtained enough rabbits to feed our family for about five days. Bev and Rhonda devised many ways of preparing rabbits for the table.

Although we spent much time at Nagambie, I was not involved in clinical medicine apart from a few notable occasions. We had a social relationship with the local doctor and I can recall on three occasions at weekends when I was working on the farm property getting a request from him to go to the hospital and help with a difficult delivery he felt was beyond his skills. After scrubbing my filthy hands well, I was able to perform a forcep delivery, thus saving the patient a trip to Shepparton by ambulance.

On one occasion during the January holiday period in the early 1970's my father and I, both at the farm property for the weekend, received a telephone request to urgently attend the Nagambie Hospital. Two young lads had been struck by a ski rope, the towing speedboat and skier passing on opposite sides of the dinghy they were fishing from. One boy was unconscious with multiple skull fractures and the other had a grossly swollen throat and difficulty in breathing. The local doctor had inserted intravenous lines and arranged an ambulance from Shepparton and police escort to transport the boys to the Royal Children's Hospital. He wanted me to come so each lad would have complete attention of a doctor while my father coped with the other patients waiting in the Emergency Department. The trip to RCH took one hour with two police cars providing escort. The boy with the injured throat required a tracheotomy prior to reaching the hospital. Both boys spent several months in hospital but survived.

~~~

Bev and I found the property at Nagambie to be a significant factor in our life. We spent time there at weekends when I was not on call and many school holidays. It was a wonderful antidote to the stress and long hours generated by my work in obstetrics and gynaecology. We developed friendships with local people and it was good for the children to be involved in some of the farm activities. Marking lambs each year involved catching and holding the lambs while they received a vaccination injection, an ear mark, a ring around their tails and for the males a ring around their scrotum. We always dined at one of the three hotels in town on Saturday night, so the children learned early in life how to behave in public.

~~~

In 1996, as part of the changes we made as we approached retirement, we sold the farm property but retained Goulburn House. We made major changes in our lifestyle which enabled us to spend more time in Nagambie, become more involved in the local community and to extend and refurbish Goulburn House and to rejuvenate the garden.

JOURNEY IN SPORT

Sport has always been a major interest to me both as an active participant and as a spectator.

As a teenager I played cricket, football and tennis at school, badminton and cricket with the Coburg Baptist Church and billiards and table tennis at home.

Whilst at University I continued to play badminton and cricket with the church and cricket with the Old Carey Grammarians. Graduation and employment in hospitals was a major impediment to sporting activities; I could not commit to play cricket as matches were played over two consecutive Saturdays and being rostered to work in the evenings made me unreliable for a badminton team.

The church had three cricket teams which played at Royal Park and Princes Park.

We played on concrete wickets covered with matting and the grounds were very rough and dusty in mid-summer. Many boys made their way to the grounds on bicycles. Bev's uncle, Horrie Dyson, had a five-ton truck and transported the matting and all the other cricket gear to the grounds each Saturday. Horrie lived in North Coburg and drove down Sydney Road to the grounds stopping to pick up many of the boys en route who would then sit on the rolls of matting loose on the tray of the truck.

Bev was the official scorer for the team for which I played.

After completing postgraduate training, I was able to arrange evening cover so could resume playing badminton, the downside being having to go back on call after returning home after midnight. Bev and I played in a team nominally from North Balwyn Baptist Church – only two of the team attended that church – until we reached our mid-fifties when various joint problems put an end to our sporting careers. Cricket was still impossible apart from occasional social matches organised at Royal Women's Hospital, obstetricians versus gynaecologists, usually won by the former.

My sporting prowess was unremarkable. I opened the bowling and batted No. 11 for the Carey First XI, made up the numbers in the First XVIII and won the billiards trophy at RWH for three consecutive years and also during my year at RCH. Bev and I were involved in a number of premiership teams in B and C Grades and won several mixed doubles titles during our badminton days.

~~~

As a spectator I followed the Richmond Football Club, attending games regularly from an early age, and have fond memories of watching players such as Jack Dyer, "Mopsy" Fraser, Ray Poulter and Roy Wright. I also spent many days at the Melbourne Cricket Ground during Test and Sheffield Shield matches.

Family commitments and medical duties played havoc with these arrangements and as the years went by, although attending the Melbourne Cricket Ground on occasions, I spent more time viewing sport on television and watching our sons play school cricket and our daughters' involvement in calisthenics and rowing.

There are several things I saw as a spectator which greatly impressed me and are worth mentioning:

- Don Bradman's last game at the MCG in December 1948 when, playing in his Testimonial Match between an XI captained by Bradman and an XI captained by Lindsay Hassett, he scored his 117th century in first class cricket. The four-day match was a tie, each team scoring 836 runs.
- Tony Ongarello played for Fitzroy in the Victoria Football League, kicking for goal with a place kick having missed several set shots earlier in the game.

- Jack Dyer of Richmond Football Club who, toward the end of his career, was handicapped by chronically damaged knees and spent much of the games in a forward pocket. When Richmond was in trouble and needed a boost he was swung into the ruck whereupon he would canter to the centre of play, run through a couple of opponents then limp back to the forward pocket. During this action spectators in the old wooden grandstand at Punt Road Oval would whistle and cheer and stamp their feet causing clouds of dust to rise out of the stand giving it the appearance of being on fire.

- Walter Lindrum, who gave an exhibition of billiards play at Coburg Town Hall. He demonstrated a vast array of difficult shots and trick shots while making an unfinished break of 600.

~~~

Active participation in competitive sport is much less prominent in the lives of young and middle-aged people today. Indeed, physical activity of any sort is less common among people of all ages, even school children. The result of this is manifest in the increasing incidence of obesity and of certain illnesses such as Type 2 diabetes and hypertension.

Gymnasiums, which were rare when I was young, are attended by people of all ages today to maintain physical fitness, important in our increasingly sedentary lifestyle. Unfortunately, few people now involve themselves in competitive sport after leaving school, particularly in team sports which have the side benefit of fostering strong inter-personal relationships and loyalty among members of the team.

JOURNEY IN MOTORING

I learned to drive at the age of 11 years in a Fargo utility, a rather basic vehicle with three forward gears, a column gear shift and no synchromesh on first gear. My teacher was Campbell O'Day, manager of the Nagambie property, who had been a transport driver during World War Two and whose opening words to me were 'people get killed in vehicles if they do silly things'. He taught me to keep both hands on the steering wheel, to drive carefully and to use the gears to decelerate as well as to accelerate; these lessons influence my driving to this day. I did a lot of supervised driving in my mother's Peugeot 203 and in my father's Nash, both of course having a manual gear shift. I also did much unsupervised driving at Nagambie in the farm utility, motorcycle and Chamberlain tractor. I did not attend a driving school and I obtained my driving licence at the age of 18 years, driving the Peugeot with my father sitting in the rear seat engaging the examiner in conversation.

Mother updated to a Wolsely in 1958 and I inherited the Peugeot. Underpowered, with a 1290cc engine and a steering column gear shift, it had some features not present in modern cars: an external switch for the rear parking lights as it was illegal to park in the street at night without a parking light showing, a crank handle which I found useful when my finances did not allow me to immediately replace a flat battery and an illuminated trafficator arm which popped out of the central pillar to indicate when turning. The latter feature was superfluous as legally one had to give hand signals when stopping or turning. Several years later flashing turning indicators became mandatory and I had these fitted: the auto-electrician did not disconnect the trafficator arms and they popped in and out in a demented fashion in time with the flashes. The Peugeot lacked many basic features of modern cars: radio, heating, cooling, and demisting. Nevertheless it was reliable, and Peter Stevenson and I did a lot of touring in the car taking our camping gear in the rather small trunk.

My second car was a Chrysler Valiant AP5, a wedding present from my parents. Roomy, and much more powerful than the Peugeot, it served us well until we went to England in 1969. Children's car seats did not exist, and the children sat in plastic seats which hooked over the back of the car seat with a fitting which could have been made from Number 8 fencing wire, or sat unrestrained on the rear central arm rest.

We spent four months in Port Moresby in 1968 as one of a series of senior registrars from the Royal Women's Hospital who spent time at the General Hospital as part of their postgraduate training. The first of these doctors had purchased a very second-hand Volkswagon Beetle which was handed to the next in line for $50 less than the predecessor had paid. I cannot recall any owners' certificate or registration papers and suspect, in retrospect, that it may have been unregistered and was certainly uninsured as it passed through the hands of a dozen different 'owners' each of whom had it for four months.

We travelled to England in 1969 and all we could afford was a second-hand Morris Minivan. An ex-Rank Xerox vehicle it was bright green and white, and the rear compartment lacked side windows. The three children travelled loose in the back. We toured much of the south of England in this vehicle during the 18 months we resided in London and, on tour, managed to fit a collapsible cot, our clothes and other essentials in the rear compartment with the children perched on top.

We returned destitute to Melbourne in 1970. Fortunately, my youngest sister Valerie was doing her nursing training and had a placement which did not allow her to use her car for several months. I borrowed it and, in those months, managed to save enough to purchase a VW 1500 Beetle. I drove this for three years then was able to update to a Peugeot 504, the first of three that served me well over the next 16 years. The second, a diesel powered sedan with manual gear shift was economical to run but very slow to accelerate; overtaking another vehicle on a country road required a different technique using a long run-up to gain momentum. I recall driving one of my friends in this car and being asked to put my foot down so that he could see what it could do; I replied that I did have my foot down. All four of our children learned to drive in this car. It had a very unsophisticated common rail diesel engine and sounded very like a Fordson tractor. Our neighbours often commented that they heard the car during the night as I drove to the hospital to deal with an emergency situation.

In 1990 I changed allegiance from Peugeots to Subaru Liberty station wagons, a change I have never regretted. The second of these, 12 years old and having travelled 180 thousand kilometres including much heavy towing, was recently replaced by a Subaru Forester.

Bev who spent time driving children around, has always had a much larger vehicle. She has driven a Morris 1500 sedan, then Ford Falcon, Holden, and Chrysler Regal station wagons. When the children had all left home, she was able to downsize to a Mitsubishi Verada sedan and currently drives a Holden Calais.

Interestingly my attitude towards motor vehicles is quite different to that of my father. He changed his car every two or three years and tended to purchase more up-market models. Among others I can recall him owning a Nash, De Soto, Jaguar, Peugeot 404 and 504, Humber Super Snipe, Vauxhall, Wolseley, Nash Rambler, Ford Fairlane and Volvo.

~~~

People frequently complain about the state of the roads, but they are infinitely better than they were in my youth. I can recall the Hume Highway as a single lane in each direction and on holiday weekends being so crowded that the normal two-hour drive from Coburg to Nagambie would take four hours. The Spirit of Progress, running between Melbourne and Sydney, crossed the Hume Highway at Craigieburn and the heavy wooden gates would be shut manually by the railway attendant about ten minutes before the train went through resulting in a queue of cars half a mile long. The speed limit on highways was the same as it is now so motorists with a closing speed of 120 mph (200 km/h) were separated by two or three metres and an interrupted white line. Towns were not by-passed and there was frequently major congestion at Kilmore as motorists sought a parking spot to break their journey. The police commonly set up speed traps in the country towns.

Modern cars are far more comfortable, more reliable, and safer than the cars of the 1950's. The cars of my youth lacked seat belts, airbags, heating and air-conditioning and often radios. They lacked current safety features such as design aimed at minimising damage to the passenger cell in the case of an accident, autonomous emergency braking, lane departure warning, rear view cameras, parking sensors and automatic lights and windscreen wipers. Automatic gear change was very rare and only available on the most expensive vehicles. Break-downs were more common than they are today; it was unusual to make the two-hour drive to Nagambie without seeing a car stationary by the side of the road with the driver changing a tyre or tinkering with the engine. Conversely the cars of the 1950's had more character than the cars of today, were more fun to drive and were much easier and cheaper to repair.

During my 62-year motoring journey I have had one significant crash when I ran into the rear of a car which unexpectedly stopped in front of me on the ramp leading onto the Eastern Freeway; no one was hurt but my Peugeot sustained considerable front end damage. I have been fined three times for speeding and breathalysed at least 20 times, passing on each occasion.

JOURNEY IN FINANCE

Doctors-in-training receive little information about financial matters nor information about organising and running a medical practice.

In the 1960s, postgraduate trainees worked long hours and were poorly paid. As a result, we were forced to live frugally and were carrying a sizeable debt when I finally completed my postgraduate training.

I commenced private practice in 1970 and considered it marvellous to earn a taxable income of $15,800 until I received a tax bill for $12,470, this being tax for the year 1970-71 of $6,235 with an equivalent amount to be pre-paid for the following year, in effect an interest free loan to the Federal Treasury. This iniquitous Provisional Tax continued to be a problem for a number of years necessitating an annual trip to the bank manager to arrange a loan to enable it to be paid.

My accountant, Mr Russell Fellow-Smith was very conservative and this, together with my own innate conservatism and ignorance of financial matters, ensured that I did not fall into the trap awaiting many young specialists of investing in tax minimisation schemes promoted by companies pushing agricultural products such as pine trees, blue gums, Wagyu cattle and Alpacas, many of which failed to provide the expected profits and taxation advantages.

The only tax-saving measure available to me was to pay Bev a significant salary for her work of being responsible for answering the work telephone between 5.00pm and 9.00am on weekdays and at weekends, working one day a fortnight in my consulting rooms and typing accounts and some letters. The Taxation Department was happy to accept this as a legitimate business expense provided the salary was not used for day to day living expenses. This enabled Bev to build up a bank balance which was put towards retirement.

The farm property at Nagambie was a commercial operation and while it did not produce a large profit neither was it helpful from the point of view of tax minimisation.

~~~

Obstetrics and gynaecology are the most poorly remunerated of all medical specialities. When the Commonwealth Department of Health was arranging the Medical Benefit Schedule in the 1960's enquiries were made regarding the fees being charged at that time by private practitioners. It is my understanding that the obstetric and gynaecology specialists asked were several conservative senior people with large private practices who charged relatively low fees. This resulted in the recommended fee structure for obstetric and gynaecology procedures being set at a low level.

There are four methods of pricing clinical services provided by medical specialists to their private patients:

- The Government Recommended Fee (or Schedule Fee) is the fee suggested by the Commonwealth Department of Health in the Medical Benefits Schedule as being appropriate for the service provided. Medicare will pay 85% of this fee. The patient is responsible for the gap between the Schedule Fee and the Medicare Rebate unless their private health care insurance provider (such as Medibank or Bupa) agrees to contribute towards the difference.

- The doctor may elect to accept the Medicare Rebate as full payment for the service and bill the Government directly (Bulkbilling) in which case the patient has no out-of-pocket expense.

- The Australian Medical Association fee schedule is the fee recommended by the AMA as appropriate and is 20-30% higher than the Schedule Fee.

- Finally, the doctor is at liberty to charge whatever fee he or she thinks is appropriate for the service provided.

It was my custom to charge the Government Recommended Fee to most patients. When I commenced practice, it was usual to charge the Medicare Rebate Fee to doctors, doctor's wives and the wives of ministers of religion and I continued to do this.

Our experience with financial advisors was mixed. Early in my career I developed a good relationship with an advisor employed by AMP who provided appropriate advice in the areas of life assurance and income protection insurance, both of great importance to a sole practitioner with a young family, and of superannuation. Unfortunately, his advice after I retired from practice was not helpful and of dubious legality and we parted ways. We attempted to develop a relationship with two other organisations offering financial advice; one gave good initial advice then suggested frequent unnecessary expensive reviews and the other gave initial advice that was not at all helpful.

Apart from the house we lived in, Bev and I had a philosophy of never making a purchase we were unable to immediately completely finance. We never leased motor vehicles as we did not wish to finance the profit made by the company arranging the lease. We used a credit card but ensured that we paid it off in full each month to avoid interest payments.

While I was working, Bev and I certainly had a comfortable lifestyle although we were not able to drive up-market cars nor take frequent expensive holidays. Interestingly we are probably better placed financially in retirement partly due to decreased expenses but mostly due to careful planning during earlier years.

JOURNEY IN RELIGION

My family began attending the Coburg Baptist Church in 1946, after we moved from the surgery premises to live in Coburg. Prior to this we had patronised either the Kew Baptist Church, which my parents had attended since childhood, or the local Brunswick Baptist Church.

The church was to have a great influence on my life, indeed, as a teenager it was the centre of my social and sporting activities. There were many families with young children and the Sunday School was attended by 70 to 80 boys and girls who also attended the morning church service. Some attended Junior Christian Endeavour on Sunday afternoon and the Sunday evening service. There was a full program of social and sporting activities. Boy's gymnasium and girl's calisthenics and the young people's social club for those older than 13 years were all well attended. There were three cricket teams which played competitively at Royal Park and Princes Park on Saturday afternoons and met for practice once during the week. There were two badminton teams, members practicing on Friday nights and playing competitively on other nights. There were tennis courts used for social but not for competitive play. Importantly there were many adults who were interested in, and took part in, these activities and who were important role models for the youngsters in the church community.

The bonding between members of the Young People's Social Club was strong and enduring. Today, 65 years later, there are some who see each other on a weekly basis and many on an occasional basis. I can readily name some 60 members of the group and note with interest that there were ten marriages, eight of them enduring, among those 60 members.

The religious instruction we received at Sunday School can be summarised in three basic tenets:

- Firstly, the Golden Rule; 'do unto others as you would have them do to you'.

- Secondly, Creation as expounded in the book of Genesis neatly summarised in the popular hymn:

> *All things bright and beautiful*
> *All creatures great and small*
> *All things wise and wonderful*
> *The Lord God made them all*
>
> *Each little flower that opens*
> *Each little bird that sings*
> *He made their glowing colours*
> *He made their tiny wings*
>
> *The purple headed mountain*
> *The river running by*
> *The sunset and the morning*
> *That brightens up the sky*
>
> *The tall trees in the greenwood*
> *The meadows where we play*
> *The rushes by the water*
> *We gather every day*
>
> *He gave us eyes to see them*
> *And lips that we might tell*
> *How great is God Almighty*
> *Who has made all things well*

- Finally, the word of Jesus Christ reported in the Gospel according to St. John – 'For God so loved the world that He gave His only begotten Son, that whosoever believeth in Him should not perish, but have everlasting life'.

Having been introduced to this doctrine at an early age we were happy to accept it uncritically, particularly in view of the fact that the church provided us with a happy social life and we were well looked after by the adult congregation. Indeed, many of us were baptised at the age of 13 or 14 indicating that we accepted these teachings.

It was during mid-teenage years that I started to think critically about these matters. I can recall some long conversations with the minister Rev. Tudball-Smith along the lines that it seemed most unfair that only those who believed in God would have eternal life when so many of the world's population had never heard of the Christian religion and had no possible chance of believing in God. Later, access to knowledge provided by geologists about the formation of the Earth and the time of appearance of plant and animal life together with the recognition of the work of Charles Darwin and others regarding the principles of Evolution, led to a re-think about matters which had seemed straight forward at Sunday School. How could one believe the Creation story as described in the book of Genesis as occurring in six days about ten thousand years ago when the world had been in existence for 13 billion years, fossils indicated life has been present for 500 million years, and our species, Homo Sapiens, has existed for 200,000 years?

Access to and consideration of this information has led me to completely revise my thoughts about religion. Information about the development of species and changes in their form in response to alterations in climate and other environmental conditions which stimulate the change, together with knowledge of the enormous length of time available for these changes to occur, make the concept of Evolution (survival of the fittest leading to improvement in a species over time) an attractive option to

Creation; nor is there need to postulate a supernatural guiding hand. The biggest, strongest, smartest, and most attractive are more likely to survive and pass on their DNA, leading to improvement of the species and even modifications leading to appearance of a new species.

My thoughts have become crystallised over the years in the following way. While it is obvious that our physical characteristics are inherited from our parents there is good evidence that our parents DNA also contributes in a major way to our mental, emotional, and possibly our spiritual makeup. However, these components of our being are also partially, indeed possibly mainly, the product of the information and guidance we receive from the many people who have an influence on our development: importantly our parents, but also others with whom we have significant contact – school teachers, relatives, friends, neighbours, our contemporaries and co-workers. This concept is neatly summarised in the African proverb – 'It takes a village to raise a child'. We owe a debt of gratitude to the society which moulded us, and it is appropriate that we repay this debt in a meaningful way. Few of us have the opportunity or the talent to make a large contribution in the way that, for instance, Fred Hollows has to the eye health of many people and particularly to those in disadvantaged communities. However, we can all make a difference to our community by living our lives according to the essential values expounded by Jesus Christ who, I believe, should be regarded as having been a wise counsellor and a gifted communicator who promoted the values of love, compassion, respect and support for others, honesty and egalitarianism. Christianity does not have a mortgage on these values; they can be equally well demonstrated by Buddhists, Hindus, Muslims, and Atheists.

To summarise my theology; a Christian is one who attempts to live his or her life according to the values expounded by Jesus Christ but has no special advantage over those who adopt the same values without attributing them to Jesus Christ. The Old Testament is a collection of books written by important Jewish leaders documenting their thoughts about the creation of the world and the history of Israel and of the Jewish people over some 500 years commencing from the time of Abraham. While it contains some marvellous poetry in the Book of Psalms I have difficulty finding relevance to me in the 20th and 21st Centuries. The New Testament written by followers of Jesus Christ is a different matter. Today, He would probably be regarded cynically by some as a knowledgeable, left-wing Jewish Rabbi with a gift for oratory. His philosophy, as mentioned before, of love, compassion, respect and support for others, honesty and egalitarianism is, if followed, guaranteed to make society a better place.

During my lifetime I have attended church regularly and estimate that I have listened to at least 3,000 sermons; I can confidently attest that none have made a measurable difference to my life. Why then attend church? The simple answer is that it is a habit; but more importantly it has enabled me to cultivate deep and enduring friendships with a wide range of people, to be involved in sporting and social activities with compatible people, and to contribute to the community by being involved in and contributing to social welfare programs.

~~~

There has been a remarkable decrease in church attendance and interest in religious matters during my lifetime, increasingly so in the last 40 years. Most Christian churches, of all denominations, have been similarly affected. It is rare nowadays to find a church which has an associated Sunday School. Some suburban churches are closing because of decreasing membership with the remaining parishioners electing to attend a nearby still functioning church, often of a different denomination, or ceasing to attend worship services at all. Many churches with ageing congregations have part-time ministers and the spiritual and social programs they offer are much less active.

The reasons for these changes are many. Some, such as Sunday sport and a wide range of activities, entertainment, and retail opportunities, together with increased mobility leading to a greater ability to enjoy them, are factors which the Church cannot control.

Better education has led to people questioning fundamental religious tenets. Theology based on the concept of an all-powerful God who created the world and everything within it and whose son, Jesus Christ, was born to Mary, a virgin who was found to be with child through the Holy Spirit, is not found attractive by better educated people who today are taught at school to question and critically examine contentious issues. The concept of Heaven and of life everlasting for believers is not enticing when one considers that at least 60% of the world's population are not Christians.

Other factors are of the Church's making. The negative publicity, heavily promoted by the media, generated because of physical, emotional and sexual mistreatment of children in orphanages and other institutions under the supervision of the Church, and even within the framework of everyday church activities has caused some people to turn away from religion. Equally as harmful has been the Church's response to this criminal treatment of children, sometimes moving miscreants to other areas, wrongly denying liability, and offering inadequate compensation to sufferers.

This problem, of the churches declining significance, can only be overcome by the Church examining and modifying its underlying theology – probably an impossible task.

There is no doubt in my mind that the Church has, despite its faults and the complexity of the theology it expounds, been a powerful force for good in the community. Is it possible that it can regain this position in the future? I am not optimistic that this will occur but think that a good starting point would be a change in emphasis to promote the virtues of respect, compassion, honesty and support for others, with less emphasis on the so-called miracles performed by Jesus Christ and the promise of eternal life for true believers. A strong stand, made in a highly visible and co-ordinated way, by all denominations, against some of the issues which lead to or result from injustice and irregularity in our society would be a good place to start. Such a stand might cause the Church to be recognized as a force for good and make it attractive to people who currently see it in a negative light. Issues which quickly come to mind include homelessness, racial intolerance, treatment of refugees and asylum seekers, the widening gulf between rich and poor members of society and business practices that are dishonest or, even if technically legal, immoral.

JOURNEY WITH FAMILY

My journey with family can be considered in three parts; the first from birth to 24 years encompassing primary, secondary, and tertiary education; the second from 24-53 years includes the years of postgraduate study, full-time work and child rearing; the third the years of diminishing workload and retirement.

~~~

The early part of my journey with family has been alluded to in earlier chapters. Suffice it to say that I was raised in a stable loving environment by parents who were honest, hard-working and religious and who both made an active contribution to their community. They were careful to 'do the right thing' and tried hard not to embarrass or cause distress to others. They were calm people not given to showing emotion. Other role models were people from the Coburg Baptist Church who tended to have a similar outlook on life.

Unfortunately, the age difference between my sisters Kathleen (Kate), five years, and Valerie, ten years, and I was too large for us to have a close relationship as children although we have become closer as the years have passed.

Society was much less complicated in those early years than it is today and there were fewer distractions. The absence of television and social media resulted in young people seeking entertainment in the areas of books, cinema, and involvement in sporting activities. It was much easier for one to decide on a career path and to pursue that path knowing that one would be able to obtain employment in the chosen area. I cannot recall being offered illicit drugs and alcohol was not taken by any in my circle of friends. However, many of us smoked tobacco and it was not until much later that this was recognised as a health hazard.

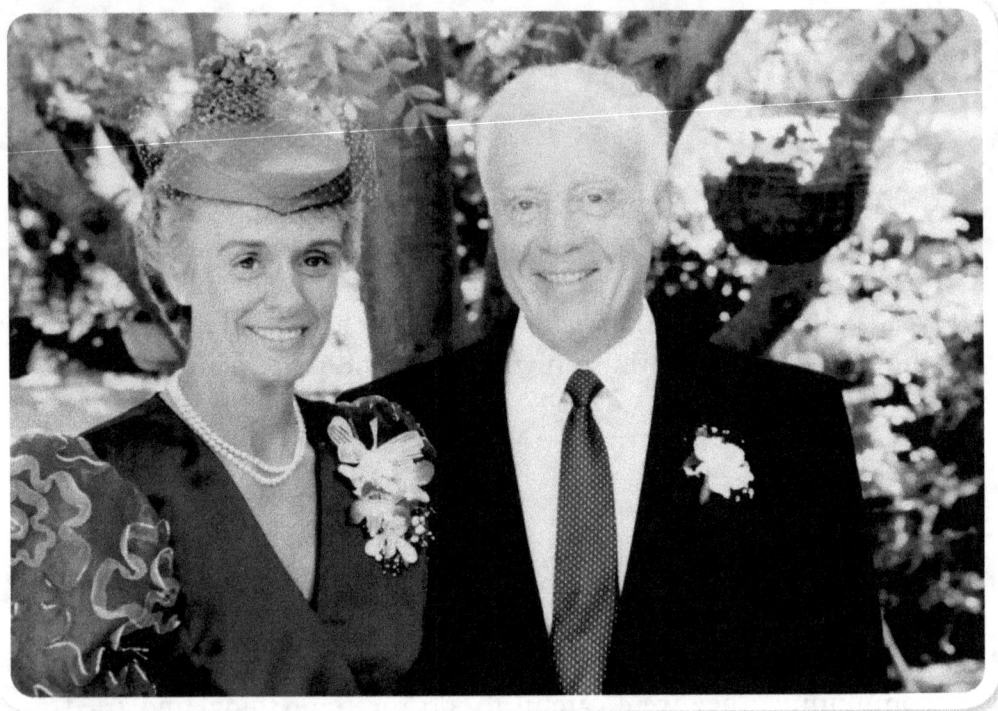

Bev and I met at Coburg Baptist Church Sunday School at the age of ten years. We attended Sunday School and Church and joined the Young People's Social Club as teenagers and became an item in our mid-teenage years. Our relationship continued during the years of secondary and tertiary education, and we married on 20th December 1963 shortly after I graduated in medicine and Bev completed her midwifery training. Our relationship has been highly successful partly due to the common interests we share, but largely because of two attributes Bev has, of being multi-skilled and self-reliant. These talents have been a major factor in our ability to cope with the stresses that accompany a busy obstetric and gynaecology practice. Prior to studying general nursing and midwifery at Bethesda Salvation Army Hospital Bev had been employed as a machinist by a firm making up-market ladies' apparel and, after studying office procedure, typing and Pitman's shorthand at Stott's Business College, had worked as a secretary and personal assistant.

Bev and I shared a common interest in sporting activities, Bev being involved in netball, athletics and calisthenics and I with football and cricket. As teenagers we both played badminton competitively and this continued until our mid-fifties when joint problems forced us, reluctantly, to abandon this activity. We shared a common interest in music, Bev as a pianist and singer and me as an observer who enjoyed most musical genres but who had no skill as a performer. These common interests in sport and music, together with our professional interests, were major factors in our ability to support each other in our married life.

~~~

Following a two-week honeymoon in Adelaide we moved into a small, sparsely furnished, upstairs single bedroom apartment in Molesworth Street, Kew. We purchased a Hoover twin-tub washing machine which set-up such a vibration that the residents of the apartment below were concerned that damage might be done to the building. I commenced work at the Royal Melbourne Hospital with a roster that required me to sleep at the hospital four nights per week. Bev stayed at the hospital some nights but the spartan resident medical officer's quarters were not conducive to dual occupancy on a regular basis. Bev worked at a local hospital but decided that her time would be better spent producing babies. Kevin was born in March 1965 to be followed 18 months later by Andrew, then 18 months later by Janine.

Kevin's birth necessitated a move to a two-bedroom apartment in Liddiard Street, Hawthorn and, in 1966, we moved into a three-bedroom two-storey house in Faraday Street in Carlton adjacent to the Royal Women's Hospital where we lived for three years. Life became more organised although the long hours on call did mean that Bev had to continue to bear most of the load of raising the children.

A close relationship developed between the doctors-in-training at RWH. There was a strong sense of community with much interaction between families. The wives joined together socially, and the children played together and, when old enough, attended kindergarten in the university precinct. A weekly highlight was Sunday lunch when all family members ate together in the doctor's dining room at the hospital.

In the 1960's women giving birth were encouraged to stay in hospital for seven days to recover from the ordeal, to bond with the baby and to establish breast feeding, a notable contrast to the situation which pertains today. After Janine's birth in 1968 Bev was able to re-waken her typing skills during the seven days of rest and type the 250-page Case Record and Commentary book which had to be assessed before I could sit the examination for entry to the Royal College of Obstetricians and Gynaecologists.

A pleasant interlude was the four months we spent in Port Moresby, TPNG, where I worked at the Port Moresby General Hospital and where a houseboy gave Bev a respite from housework apart from shopping, preparation of meals and, of course, breast feeding Janine. Kevin and Andrew enjoyed the company of the house-boy and were disappointed when Tuna could not accompany us back to Melbourne.

We returned to RWH for a further four months until my term of employment ceased in March 1969 and we had to vacate the house in Faraday Street. We had no property of our own in which to live. I had to sit for the MRCOG examination in six weeks and we were booked to sail to England in eight weeks. Bev and the children went to Nagambie to live with my sister Kate while I lived weekdays with my parents and studied for the examination and spent weekends in Nagambie – not an ideal situation and very tough for Bev.

Eventually the time passed, I was successful in the examination, and we boarded the Greek registered liner *Australis* for the trip to England. This was a further difficult time as the children, one by one in order of seniority, developed measles. In those pre-vaccination times measles was endemic on ships with their changing population and with children in close proximity to each other. Bev's nursing skills were invaluable as Janine was particularly sick with high fever and signs suggestive of mild encephalitis. Fortunately, there was a paediatrician I knew aboard the ship, and he was able to confirm that we were doing all that was possible to care for Janine and she made a good recovery. Having recovered from the measles onslaught the children proceeded, one by one, to develop chicken pox, Janine's rash appearing as we disembarked at Southampton.

Fortunately, we had arranged a week's accommodation in a London hotel through the Overseas Visitors Club where Bev cared for the ailing children while I made contact with West Middlesex Hospital where I was to work, found accommodation nearby and purchased a second-hand Morris Minivan.

We moved into a three-bedroom house in Whitton, next door to a couple with two daughters of similar age to our children. The low trellis fence between the two back yards was demolished to make one large play area. Jackie and John Newnham became firm friends, and the two families spent much time together.

We spent many weekends exploring London with its famous buildings and landmarks and enjoyed Richmond Park, Kew Gardens and Hampton Court Palace which were nearby. The long summer evenings were particularly enjoyable, and we frequently took a picnic lunch or tea to one of the many parks.

We enjoyed short breaks away at Yarmouth and Norfolk and had one week at Billy Butlin's Holiday Camp at Torquay, Devon, the latter entailing a 180-mile drive which took eight hours as we travelled on a bank holiday.

Kevin commenced school and developed an English accent. The children were provided with a midday meal; the first he had was stew and salad which he described to us as being 'dog meat and grass'. He frequently played with a school friend who lived nearby whose father complained that his son was starting to develop an Australian accent.

I was on call three nights a week at WMH and shared the duty officer's bedroom with a female Persian registrar. The room was frequently festooned in drying items of female apparel, and I was uncertain as to whether the bed linen was changed each day so elected to take the night calls from home, only ten minutes from the hospital. This arrangement worked well and enabled me to spend much more time with the family.

Winter was challenging with daylight lasting from 9.00am until 3.30pm. Unusually for London we saw seven falls of snow and Bev has vivid memories of trudging through the snow with Janine and Andrew in a pusher and Kevin walking beside her as she took him to and from school in the dark or went shopping. Andrew caused some embarrassment on one these shopping expeditions – left briefly in the foyer of the supermarket he drew much attention by loudly singing the current Rolf Harris hit *I've Lost My Mummy*.

There were several fellow travellers also obtaining postgraduate experience, mostly in provincial hospitals. They stayed with us when they visited London and it was common to have three or four children sleeping side-by-side and end-to-end in a single bed. In return this enabled us to have accommodation when we travelled north to explore Cambridge and Newcastle.

We travelled back to Melbourne in mid-1970 in a Qantas Boeing 707, a 31-hour flight with one two hour refuelling stop in Bangkok. I looked after the boys who were quiet and slept much of the time while Bev sat with Janine who was hyper-active, noisy, and slept very little – not a good trip but much better than six weeks on a ship. Our parents welcomed us at Tullamarine, and all travelled to my parent's home in East Ivanhoe where Bev and I and the children lived with my parents for six weeks. Within a week Kevin had started school at East Ivanhoe Primary School where, because of his accent, he was known as the English kid. We found a suitable house which we purchased at auction with a 10% deposit and the loan for the remainder arranged with the Commercial Bank of Australia, guaranteed by my father.

After moving into the house in Waterdale Road, Ivanhoe (the eighth residence we had occupied in seven years of marriage) we at last found some stability. The children were delighted with their new home, and we realised how they had been affected by all our moves when Kevin, sitting beside an electric heater on a cold wintry day, asked 'When we move next could we take this with us?'

Life proceeded on an unremarkable path with the children receiving their primary education at East Ivanhoe Primary School and their secondary education at Carey Baptist Grammar School apart from Janine who spent four years at Strathcona Girls Grammar School until Carey became co-educational and commenced taking girls at the appropriate level.

Nicola was born in 1971. Much smaller at birth than her siblings and very blonde, she appeared to be fragile but was, in fact, very resilient having been toughened by playing with her older siblings. Her musical ability showed itself at an early age; she was able to pick out tunes on the piano at the age of two and a half years.

My father died following a stroke in 1975 at the age of 67 years. His health had not been robust; he suffered from a duodenal ulcer which had necessitated admission to hospital and blood transfusion on several occasions and had significant arterial disease which had led to surgery for aortic and popliteal aneurisms. He and I enjoyed a close relationship, and I was devastated by his death. Bev and I made a significant mistake – because Nicola was only three years old we thought it would be best if the children did not attend the funeral. In retrospect this was wrong as it did not allow the boys, now aged nine and ten, to say goodbye to their grandfather who had been an important factor in their lives. The decisions one makes are not always correct particularly when they are made in times of emotional stress.

At the time of my father's death my parents were in the process of finalising his retirement and were planning to sell the family home at 269 The Boulevard, East Ivanhoe and move to Goulburn House in Nagambie. Fortuitously the dwelling behind the family home came on the market. We were able to purchase this smaller property for my mother and Bev and I and the children moved into the family home. This arrangement was ideal; it enabled the children to see their grandmother as they took a short cut through her property to and from primary school, facilitated by a gate installed in the dividing fence, and in later years as she became frail enabled us to check that all was well.

All four of our children successfully completed the Victorian Certificate of Education. Three completed University courses, graduating as follows:

- Kevin, MB. BS., (Melbourne).

- Janine, B.App.Sc. Physical Education,
  (Phillip Institute of Technology).
  Dip. Ed., (La Trobe).

- Nicola, B.Ed. Sec., (Melbourne).

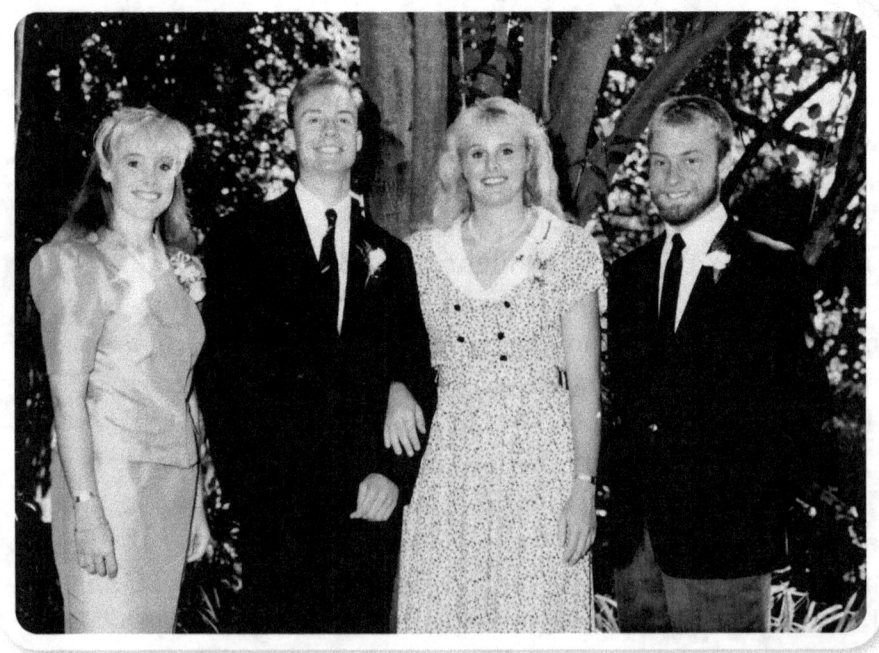

Andrew caused us some anxiety; uncertain about his future he did two years of agricultural science at La Trobe University but seeing no future in farming abandoned the course and spent some time doing labouring jobs and delivering pizzas. For several years he worked as a labourer for a landscape gardener whose main work was installing sprinkler systems in bowling greens and parks. When this business failed Andrew had learned enough about irrigation to be employed as an irrigation consultant by a local nursery. This job led to a position with a larger firm and ultimately to an appointment as manager at their Geelong and then Shepparton branches. He now owns his own business, Water Plus, in Shepparton.

After appropriate postgraduate training Kevin commenced general practice as a family doctor, initially working as an assistant and finally becoming a partner in a practice in Surrey Hills.

Janine was initially employed at Broadmeadows College where she coped well with the rather unrefined clientele attending the school. After seven years she sought employment at Blackburn High School then Balwyn High School where she continues to work as a relieving teacher in the physical education department.

Nicola's first position was music and drama teacher at Tintern Girls School and she now works as a private music teacher at Glen Katherine Primary School in the St. Helena Secondary College campus and at her home.

~~~

I commenced a prolonged retirement process detailed elsewhere in 1992. Significant changes occurred in our family life. All four children were married, Kevin to Lydia Tkach in the Ukrainian Church at Essendon, Janine to Dominic O'Shaughnessy in Xavier Chapel, Andrew to Claire Dunshea in St. Aidan's Uniting Church at North Balwyn and Nicola to Bruce Ramsay in the Kew Baptist Church. Janine's marriage failed after 18 years, and she subsequently married Neil Bone.

The first grandchild was born in 1995 to be followed by seven in the next four years and two more in the next three years. Bev and I had clearly indicated that we were not available for child minding on a regular basis but were certainly available for occasional and emergency situations. The latter situation occurred, and we were very involved in the care of our first grandchild, Larissa and her mother Lydia for six months then to a lesser degree for a further 12 months. Janine's second child Sarah, born when her sister

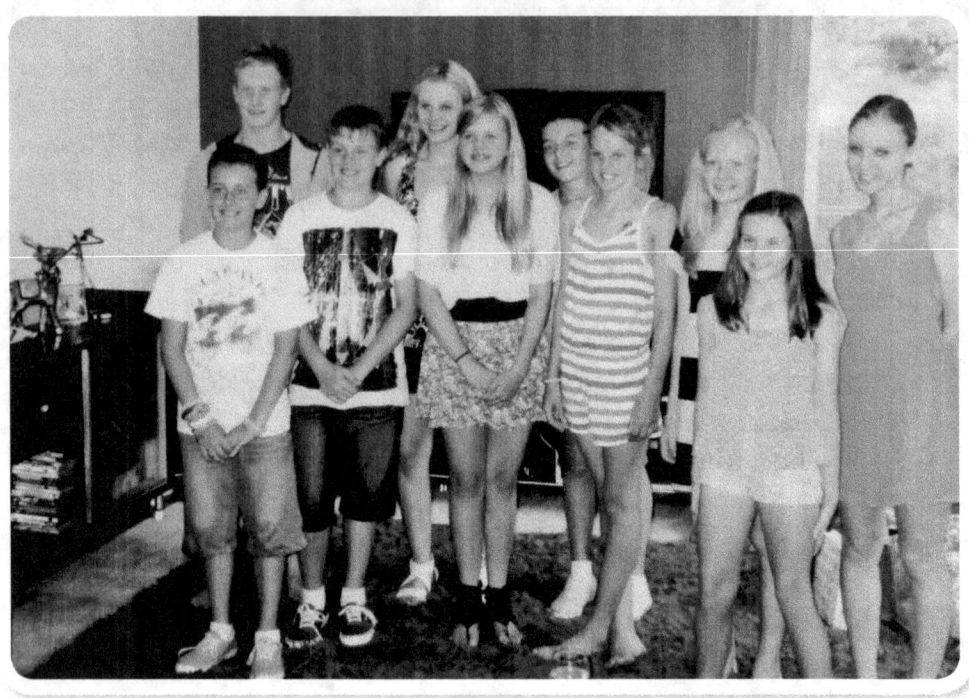

Katelyn was 16 months old, had significant physical problems which necessitated her spending much of her first nine months of life in the Royal Children's Hospital. In order to allow Janine to spend most of her time at the hospital Katelyn lived with us – certainly a change to have to care for a two-year-old 24/7 in your late fifties. It was fascinating to observe the interaction between Larissa and Katelyn separated in age by only three months.

During the succeeding years the grandchildren spent many happy times at Nagambie with us during school holidays. Being so close in age they relate well to each other, and firm bonds of friendships were formed. They spent most of their time outside where they involved themselves in activities such as building Heath Robinson type rabbit traps, constructing mini-golf courses, playing football, cricket and golf, and swimming in the pool.

It is very pleasing to note that all grandchildren have developed a strong work ethic. After leaving school most have been involved in part-time work while pursuing their tertiary studies. Currently of the eight who have completed secondary education, three (Katelyn, Kane and Tom) are working full time having completed or being currently involved in tertiary studies; one (Larissa) has completed a university degree in biomedicine and is working towards a PhD; three are undertaking a university degree, Sarah (nursing/psychology), Kelly (outdoor education) and Joel (computer science). Stephanie is working part-time in three different jobs while deciding where her career lies. Mitchell and Emily are still at secondary school.

~~~

The journey with family has been a fascinating one. Observing your children develop from birth, pass through the years of education during childhood and early adulthood, to become mature stable citizens making a worthwhile contribution to the community has been interesting. It is satisfying to know that one has played a part in this process. We now have the joy of seeing our grandchildren follow the same path, realising that the pitfalls besetting them are far greater than the ones that our children encountered and far, far greater than the ones that we had to negotiate.

~~~

Wikipedia defines a family as a group of people related either by birth or by marriage or other relationships. The family unit increases in size and complexity with the passage of time as the children marry and produce grandchildren who, in turn, repeat the process. This increase introduces people with different backgrounds and skill sets, a process which invigorates the family unit. The glue which binds the members of the group together are love and respect, patience, and tolerance.

Human beings are social creatures and derive much pleasure from the companionship and support they receive from their relatives. Another of the joys of belonging to a family group is the ability to remember and reminisce about events that have occurred in the past, particularly when the children are young. I have alluded to some of these in earlier chapters but feel it appropriate to consider some others:

- Kevin walked unaided at nine months of age and was able to pass unimpeded under a table. As he grew taller it took a little time for him to realise that he could no longer do this without bumping his head.

- Kevin aged three years, playing happily in a sandpit I constructed from recycled timber and filled with sand procured from Brighton Beach. He came into the house one day proudly 'smoking' a cigarette butt he had found in the sand.

- Andrew aged two, talking fluently and asking the question 'Why?' incessantly. My parents frequently took the boys with them to Nagambie for the weekend. Andrew, sitting on the rear central arm rest (there were no car seats in those days), would talk endlessly during the two hour drive prompting my father to ask my mother 'Doesn't that kid ever shut up?'

- In the 1960's it was fashionable for women to wear hats to church. Bev was forced to abandon this practice when Andrew, aged 18 months, repeatedly removed her hat, and placed it on his own head.

- The children learned the correct anatomical names for body parts at an early age, for example clavicle for collar bone and scapula for shoulder blade. Janine, aged two and a half years, watching a friend of ours change the nappy of her newborn baby, observed to the mother that it was a boy baby because it had a penis. In similar vein as Bev approached full term with Nicola, Janine would follow her to the toilet and stand at the door warning her not to drop the baby in the toilet.

- Andrew at four-year-old kindergarten show and tell related that he had spent the previous weekend at Nagambie and had helped 'mark the calves' and that this involved 'crushing their scrotums'.

- Bev isolating herself in the children's playpen to iron the clothes while they had the run of the house.

- Janine, aged two and a half years, sustained a spiral fracture of the tibia while playing a rough game with her brothers. Green whistles were not available so I gave her an injection of Pethidine before driving her to my father's surgery where we confirmed the diagnosis with x-ray, then applied a plaster from mid-thigh to the toes to immobilise the fracture. She 'bottom-hopped' for two days then walked in the plaster necessitating that it be reinforced. When the plaster was removed eight weeks later, she screamed loudly when grandpa approached with the plaster shears thinking that he was going to cut her leg off. She walked with a stiff leg after removal of the plaster; a problem that was cured by taking her to the beach to swim and play on the sand.

- Janine enjoyed primary school so much so that each day, on returning home, she sat Nicola, aged three years, in front of a small blackboard and passed on the knowledge that she had acquired.

- Andrew in grade four was told by his teacher that he would not be allowed to graduate from a pencil to a pen until his writing improved. His response – 'I won't write better until I have a pen!'

- Nicola, younger than the other children interfered in their games at times. They dealt with this problem by locking her in a cupboard. Bev and I did not know about this until many years later.

- My parents had a very patient and long-suffering elderly Labrador. Jenny allowed the children to climb all over her. Occasionally, when their play became too rough, she would shake them off and move to another area of the garden.

- Janine aged two years, badly wanted to be a boy like her brothers! Indeed, she insisted that she was a boy and refused to wear dresses. She was very upset when her grandmother, at Christmas, gave the boys cowboy suits and gave her a cowgirl skirt and jacket – it had to be changed.

- When Bev, and the three children, lived with my sister Kate at Nagambie prior to us travelling to England we were a little concerned about their relationship with Kate's dog, a Doberman named Elka. We need not have worried. Elka became very protective of them, even rounding them up when Bev called them to come inside.

- Nicola and Janine were heavily involved in calisthenics, as was Bev who played the piano accompaniment for their weekly club practice sessions and for concerts and competitions. Kevin, Andrew, and I attended the concerts somewhat reluctantly. I arrived home from work one evening to find a scene of confusion and anxiety; Nicola, running with a calisthenics rod in her mouth, had fallen and sustained an injury to the tissue in front of her left tonsil which was bleeding freely. Control was achieved by applying firm pressure to the area for ten minutes using a pad of gauze.

- The children received their regular immunisation injections through the program organised by the Infant Welfare Centre. Some booster injections, e.g., for Tetanus, were needed after they had ceased attending the Centre and I administered these at home. Nicola was particularly nervous and vocal about this, and the situation had to be eased by bribing her with a substantial chocolate reward.

- The children note that Bev and I largely ignored their minor illnesses and that the standard treatment for most complaints was 'Take a Panadol'. They also note that, unlike many of their friends, they were never able to stay home from school by pretending to be unwell.

JOURNEY IN RETIREMENT

Two factors encouraged me to plan for early retirement from the full-time work force. Foremost was the somewhat dispiriting family history of a father who died at 67 years of age, a grandfather at 57 and a great-grandfather at 47. A second consideration was the stressful and disorganised, albeit interesting and rewarding life led by a busy obstetrics and gynaecology specialist engaged in private and public hospital clinical practice.

Many of my senior colleagues did not cope well with retirement largely because they did not have significant interests outside medicine and little contact with people other than their work mates. Fortunately, Bev and I had many interests outside medicine and most of our friends were not from the medical profession. Many medical retirees also find difficulty in coping with a sudden cessation of all medical work; a gradual decrease in the workload leading to a gentle retirement process is often not possible. Fortunately, I was able to organise a protracted retirement process.

The first step towards retirement was taken in 1992 when, at the age of 53 years, I ceased private practice but continued to work full-time in administration and clinical care of public hospital patients at RWH and MHW. The immediate effect of this was to reduce on-call weekends from one in two to one in five and to reduce weeknight on-call from five in five to one in five. I still worked about 50 hours per week, but the pace of work was much reduced. I enjoyed the administration work and was able to spend much more time teaching and counselling junior staff.

Four years later I retired from RWH, relinquishing the administrative function and care of public inpatients. My only remaining clinical responsibility was one public antenatal clinic per week at MHW which I continued until 2009 when, at the age of 70 years, I retired from all clinical work.

This gradual retirement, spread over 17 years, suited our lifestyle well and Bev and I were fortunate to be able to be involved in several different projects during this time.

RELOCATION TO NAGAMBIE

In 1998 Bev and I engineered a major change in our lifestyle. After selling the farm property in 1996 we spent more time at Goulburn House. Our four children were married and having no need for a house with five bedrooms, we sold the family home in East Ivanhoe and purchased a small property at 18 Lena Street in Viewbank. Our plan was to make Goulburn House our main dwelling, live there five days per week with two days in Viewbank, thus enabling us to continue to spend time with our three children in Melbourne and their families, to maintain existing friendships in Melbourne, to attend Probus club meetings and functions and for Bev to continue attending rehearsals with the Melbourne Chorale. We were also close to our son Andrew and his family who lived in Shepparton and were able to see them more often.

This change in lifestyle worked well and we rapidly became involved in many aspects of community life in Nagambie, further enlarging our circle of friends.

RENOVATION OF GOULBURN HOUSE

Although Goulburn House had been owned by the Ratten family since 1969 it had been used as a holiday house and little had been spent on upkeep of the home and garden.

Renovation and extension of the house was a major challenge, planned and executed brilliantly by Greg Hopkins, a carpenter and builder from the adjacent town of Avenel. The work was done in four stages; removal of decaying weatherboard additions from the rear of the house which included a laundry, bathroom, bedroom and verandah; replacing these with a complex composed of a guest wing with two bedrooms, bathroom, shower room and toilet, laundry, and a large sitting room with a dining alcove; remodelling the kitchen; and refurbishing the original part of the house. Removing the weatherboard add-ons enabled us to restore a return verandah which completely encircled the house.

The whole process took one year to complete during which time Bev and I slept in various rooms that were not being worked on at the time, washed ourselves and our clothes and prepared our meals in a bathroom. Needless to say, many evening meals were taken in one of the local hotels. In previous years a detached rumpus room had been built but we could not live in this complex as it was full of furniture from the house being renovated.

REJUVENATION OF GOULBURN HOUSE GARDEN

Rejuvenating the garden which covered two acres was an equally demanding task. Much of the area was covered by small ill-developed peppercorn trees, briar rose, boxthorn and stunted trees Bev describes as bird droppings. There were two large pine trees at the front fence overhanging the road, both decaying and occasionally dropping branches, which needed to be removed. The local council brought in their grader and pulled the trees over so we could cut them into sections with a chain saw. A local farmer used his tractor with a grader blade to push much of the unwanted vegetation into a large heap. I then worked on the residue and, with the help of John Clarke, a local gardener, cleared the remaining rubbish vegetation adding it to the heap until it was 20 metres in diameter and two metres high. After speaking with the local CFA captain, we set fire to the heap with the fire truck parked nearby; it burned for a week.

With a blank canvas we now started to define garden beds, build arbours and paths, and planted a selection of native plants, fruit trees, bulbs, roses and a large vegetable garden which had to be securely fenced to protect it from the depredation of rabbits which are ubiquitous in Nagambie. As the garden beds were formed, we installed a sprinkler system to enable automatic watering of the extensive garden.

Like all gardens it remained a work in progress being continually modified and added to. It was a continuing source of joy to us and provided me with at least one day of moderate exercise each week. Clipping the hedges and pruning the 200 rose bushes was the most challenging part of maintenance work.

INVOLVEMENT WITH NAGAMBIE HEALTH CARE

Shortly after moving to live permanently in Nagambie, one of our friends suggested that I should join the Committee of Management of Nagambie Hospital and that Bev should join the Ladies Auxiliary. Nagambie Hospital is a Bush Nursing Hospital owned by the community and the management committee is elected by the community; at that time the committee members were owners of local small businesses, a schoolteacher, a farmer and a bookkeeper, none of whom had great knowledge of health care. In 1983 there were 38 Bush Nursing Hospitals in Victoria and they accounted for one third of the state's hospital beds. Changes in the method of funding in the 1980's and the 1990's resulted in severe financial difficulty for these institutions, and many were forced to close. Currently Nagambie is one of five still functioning.

Within four months of joining the committee it became obvious that the hospital was in a dire financial position and would need to close. To compound the problem the Chief Executive Officer, no doubt seeing the writing on the wall, had resigned several months previously. The hospital, at that time, consisted of 20 aged care beds and 15 acute hospital beds. The age care beds were always fully occupied, and although we closed the hospital, it was possible to continue operating these by placing them temporarily under the control of nearby Euroa Hospital, thus avoiding having to relocate 20 frail elderly people to accommodation in other towns.

A bush nursing hospital such as Nagambie is a vital part of the community for, as well as providing aged care accommodation, emergency care and hospital accommodation for sick people, it provides work for many local people. A community meeting was held, and the Committee of Management was instructed to endeavour to find a way to re-open the hospital. At this time the board chairman, a small business owner, decided that this would be beyond his skills and I was invited to take the position of Chairman of the Committee of Management.

Six hundred thousand dollars was raised within the Nagambie community by means of donations, several legacies, and the proceeds of two wheat crops organised by a group of farmers, the Crop Committee, who donated a paddock and their labour and arranged for donations of seed and fertilizer by agricultural suppliers. Nagambie's Commonwealth and State Government representatives were very supportive, and we received advice and generous financial assistance from both governments to the extent that we were able to spend $1.8 million refurbishing and extending the building, increasing the number of beds by 50% to make the institution financially viable. I was delighted to be awarded Life Membership of the Hospital in recognition for the work in leading the team which rescued it from closure.

Since it re-opened, Nagambie HealthCare has gone from strength to strength. Additional extensions have been made to further increase bed numbers and bed occupancy is always close to 100%. A multi-purpose complex has been built to house a medical clinic, a physiotherapist, and a function room. Five units have been built on the hospital site overlooking Lake Nagambie to provide accommodation for people capable of independent living who wish to live close to hospital services and there are plans to provide more of this type of accommodation.

Thus, Nagambie HealthCare has acute hospital beds and provides independent living units and low and high aged care accommodation. It also has a room dedicated to the care of patients with terminal illness. There is a medical practice on site and accommodation for ancillary health providers.

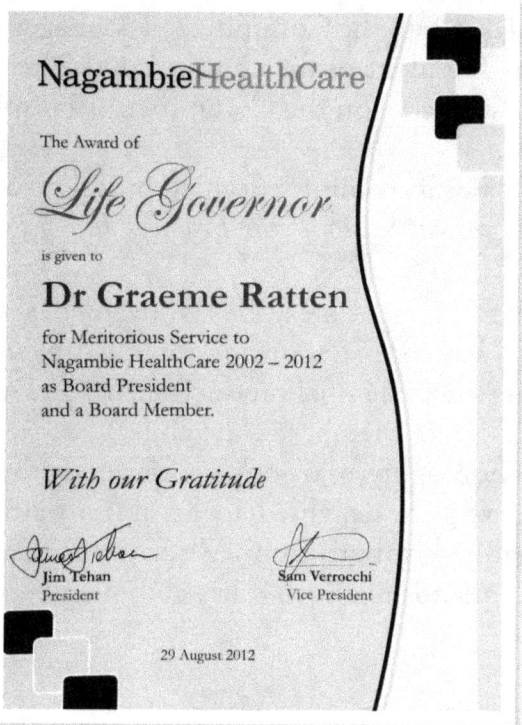

PROBUS

I joined the Probus Club of Heidelberg in June 1997. Probus is an organisation for people who want to maintain a social link with others who have similar interests and are largely or completely retired from their professional and business lives. Each Probus club is sponsored by a Rotary Club and the Probus Club of Heidelberg, sponsored by the Heidelberg Rotary Club, was formed in 1983. There is a monthly club meeting when members meet for fellowship and to enjoy a short talk given by a club member on a subject of his choice (Member's corner) and an address by an external Guest Speaker. The club also arranges monthly outings to a local point of interest together with a lunch and, during most years, organises a five-day trip to a Victorian rural centre or a 10 day trip to an overseas venue. Some of the earlier established clubs, such as the Heidelberg Probus club or the Rosanna Ladies Probus Club, to which Bev belongs, are single sex clubs; more recently clubs are required to be open to people of both genders.

I was invited to join the Committee of Management in March 1998 and was President of the club in 2000-2001 and again in 2005-2006. I still serve on the Committee as Hospitality Officer and Historian.

I was part of a sub-committee which produced a 70-page club history, *An Historical Salute – The Probus Club of Heidelberg – 20 Years – 1983 – 2003*.

For my work in this area, I was awarded a Certificate of Appreciation. I have been responsible for updating the club history every five years since its initial production and in December 2009 was appointed a Life Member of the club.

Bev and I thoroughly enjoy our association with our respective Probus clubs and are delighted to be able to attend functions and trips organised by both clubs. We have made many firm and long-standing friendships with other club members.

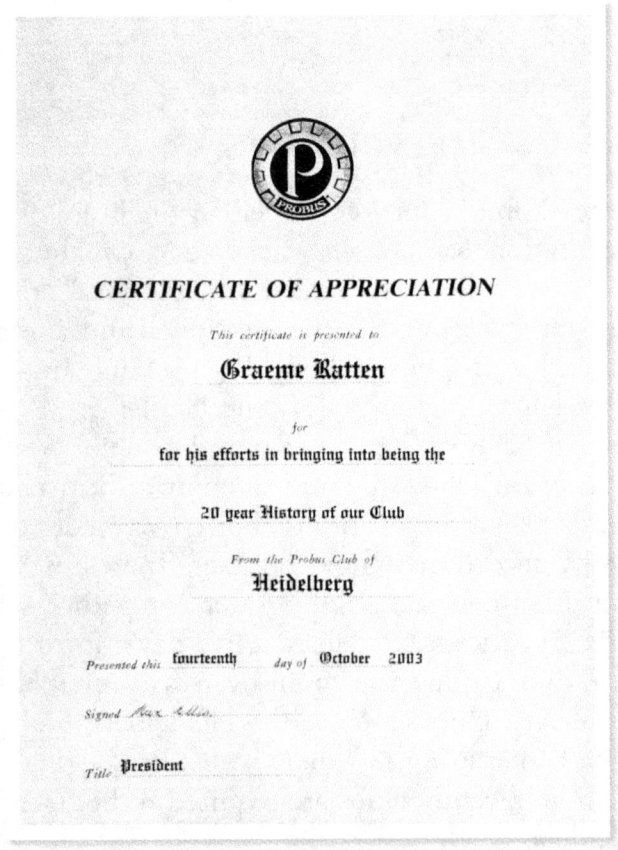

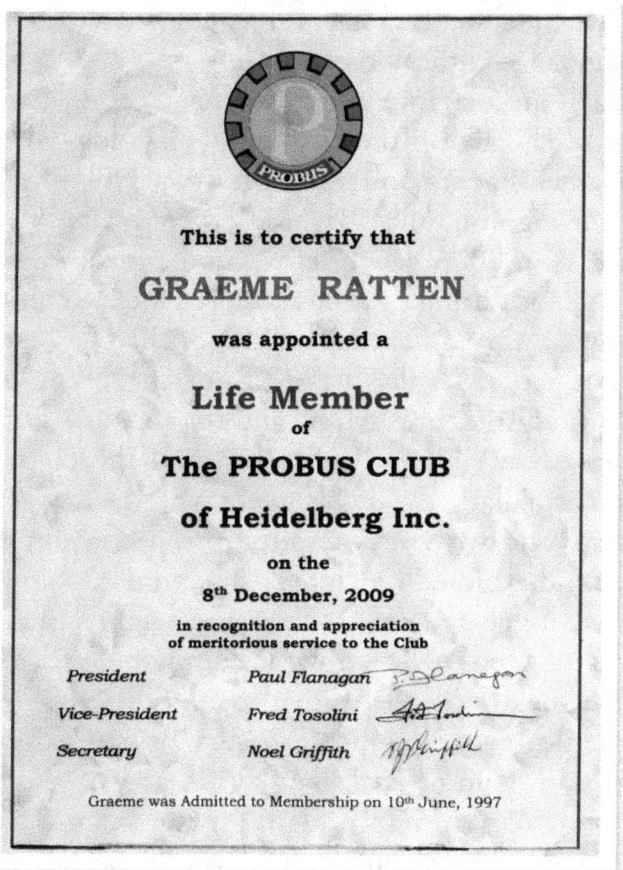

INVOLVEMENT WITH OCEANIA UNIVERSITY OF MEDICINE, SAMOA

In 2005 I met with Professor Surindar Cheema, Vice-Chancellor of OUM. There is a School of Nursing in Apia, the capital of Independent Samoa, located on the largest island, Upolo, but until the formation of OUM every Samoan wishing to study medicine attended medical school in Fiji or in Papua New Guinea and received postgraduate training in Australia or New Zealand. OUM is an initiative aimed at addressing this deficiency and is backed by American philanthropists and has a council composed of Americans and Samoans. It is a private university but native Samoans entering the course are awarded a scholarship. Fee-paying students come mainly from Australia, New Zealand and

America. Much of the teaching is done online and students spend time in Samoa for clinical instruction.

Professor Cheema invited me to review the material used for online teaching of obstetrics and gynaecology, to make any necessary amendments and to suggest ways of improving the syllabus. Having done this, Bev and I were invited to visit Apia for two weeks in 2006. My brief was to be involved in teaching medical students during their clinical placement in obstetrics and gynaecology and to assess the facilities of the National Hospital (Tupua Tamesese Meaole, TTM) from the point of view of patient care and student teaching and to provide a written report to the Vice-Chancellor of the University. I thoroughly enjoyed this work, particularly the involvement with the medical students and Bev enjoyed two weeks respite from household duties. We hired a car and explored much of the island of Upolo.

Samoa is a highly religious society. The majority of the 180,000 inhabitants of Upolo, the most heavily populated of the nine islands that make up Independent Samoa, live in villages each of which has its own church and pastor. Bev and I attended the Apia Protestant Church each Sunday where we were made very welcome and enjoyed the wonderful hymn singing provided by the church choir. Indeed, at our first visit the pastor invited us to stand, introduce ourselves and explain the reason for our visit. Following the morning church service Samoans have a family dinner and spend the afternoon together. Most retail outlets apart from convenience stores are closed on Sunday.

In 2007 I was invited back to Samoa to attend the inaugural OUM Graduation Ceremony. The ceremony for the five graduands was impressive and was held at the National University of Samoa in an enormous fale; large enough to accommodate 600 people it was built entirely of timber with a shingle roof. Speakers included the Minister of Health, Honorable Gatolocifuana Alesama-Gidlow, the Chairman of the National Council of Churches Rev. Okafoucolo, chairperson of OUM Council Mrs Taffy Gould, Vice-Chancellor Professor Surindar Cheema and the keynote speaker was Prime Minister Turleopa Sailata Maliebebgaor.

In 2009 Bev and I returned to Apia for two weeks. On this occasion I was involved in clinical teaching of medical students and was Chief Censor for the Final Clinical Examination. I was asked to review the facilities of the OUM and of the TTM hospital, on this occasion writing a report for the Deputy Dean of OUM Doctor Monalisa Punicalu. Once again, we enjoyed our time and, I think, made a significant contribution to the teaching and examining of medical students.

I made two further trips to Samoa in 2010 and 2011, on each occasion acting as an external examiner in the Final Clinical Examination.

My work in Samoa was done on an honorary basis with my fares and accommodation (and Bev's) paid by OUM and I was awarded the title of Honorary Associate Professor.

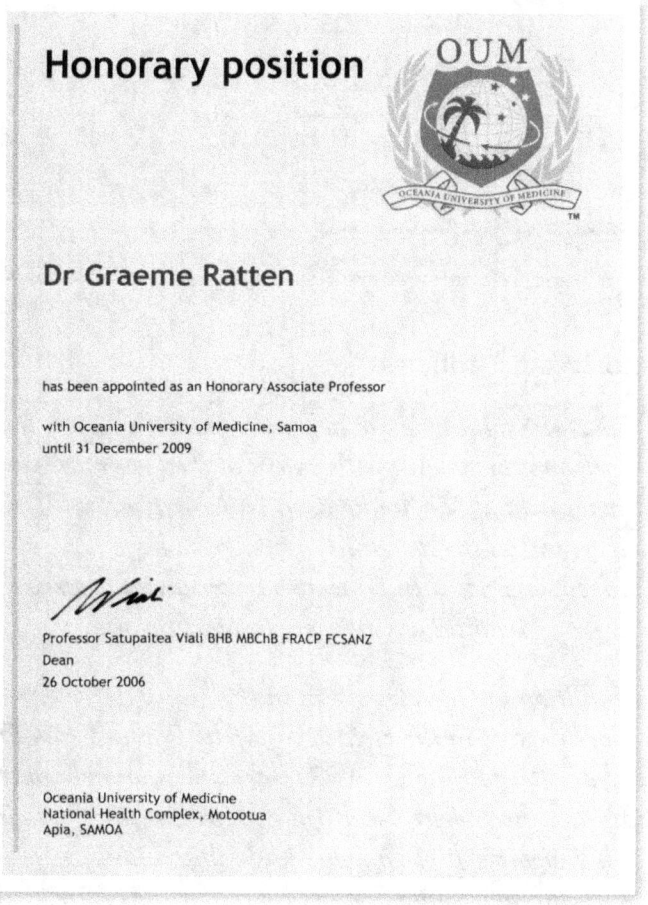

COMMUNITY AWARD

On 26th January 2008 I received a Jaga Jaga Community Australia Day Award presented by The Honorable Jenny Macklin M.P. Federal Member for Jaga Jaga.

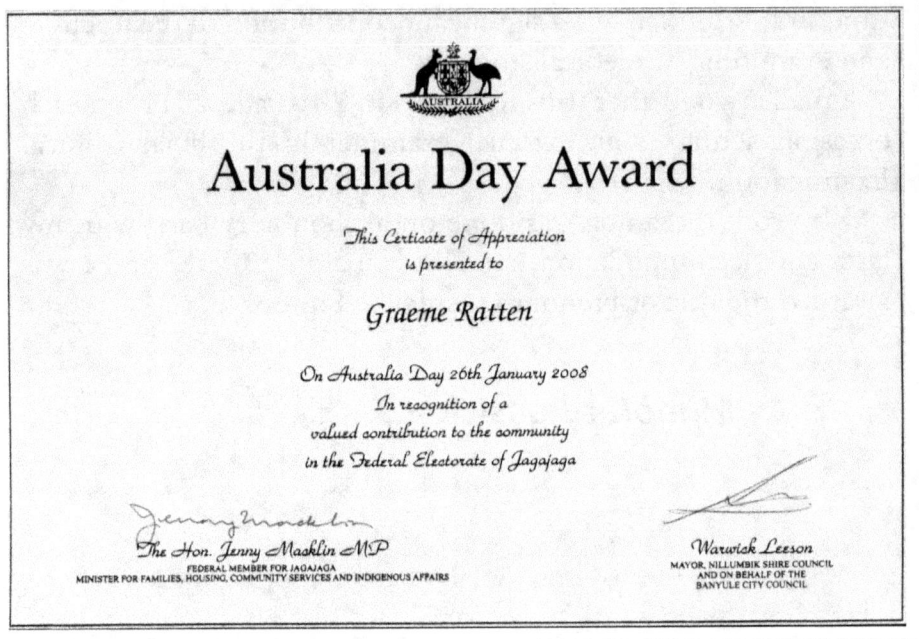

The citation read as follows:

> 'Graeme's willingness to help his community spans two different areas. As the President of the Committee of Management of Nagambie Bush Nursing Hospital Graeme was central in the successful campaign to have the hospital reopened. Since then Graeme has continued to serve the hospital as Chair of Hospital Board.
>
> In addition to Graeme's efforts in the health sector Graeme has been active in the Heidelberg Men's Probus Club. Only one year after joining in 1997 Graeme was brought onto the club's executive where he instigated a process that revitalized the club membership. Graeme's leadership skills have seen the club move onto a sound course for the future.'

TRAVEL

While I was working full-time, we were unable to take more than two weeks holiday at one time and were mostly restricted to one week. This curtailed our ability to travel overseas and even within Australia and it was not until I had commenced the retirement process that we were able to correct this anomaly.

Accordingly, during the last 20 years Bev and I have travelled overseas, sometimes with two friends from Nagambie, sometimes with Probus friends and occasionally on our own, to Europe, Canada and Alaska, the United Kingdom, Scandinavia and Russia, Vietnam, Cambodia and China, Mauritius, Borneo, New Caledonia, Norfolk Island, Lord Howe Island, New York and Hawaii, Japan, Hong Kong, and Singapore. Within Australia we have taken trips to Broome and the Kimberley, Lake Eyre, Outback Queensland, Cape York, Western New South Wales, Alice Springs and Uluru and Western Australia. With Probus we have travelled to several Victorian centres such as Barham, Hamilton and Gippsland.

We found coach travel organised by a tour company more relaxing than self-drive holidays and like the concept of being looked after, not having to decide where to eat and sleep, not having to drive, being taken to the best tourist places by a knowledgeable guide and particularly the better views one gets of passing scenery from a coach compared to a motor car.

It has been my habit to keep a diary during these ventures and on returning home to use these notes together with relevant pamphlets we collected and pictures we had taken, to produce an illustrated account of the holiday. These accounts have been used to prepare short talks which Bev and I have given at our respective Probus clubs. They are great mementos allowing us to look back and remind ourselves of the happy times we had while touring.

We have made many good friends during our travels and are especially pleased that, 15 years after a long tour through Europe, one-third of the group are able to meet every second year for a three-day reunion.

RETURN TO MELBOURNE

As we entered our eighth decade, Bev and I gave serious thought to our future lifestyle. We both enjoyed living in Nagambie, particularly the relaxed lifestyle, the great friends we had made and our involvement in community affairs. We were very happy living in Goulburn House and found upkeep of the large garden a pleasure. The two days we spent in Melbourne each week enabled us to remain involved in our Probus clubs, meet with our children and grandchildren and other friends who lived in Melbourne. However, we could see that sometime in the future problems would arise when one of us developed a physical disability that restricted our activity. We mulled this problem over for two years before making the decision to sell the Nagambie property and return to Melbourne.

Selling the property was easy compared to the task of emptying the house of contents accumulated over 45 years. The Salvation Army and local Opportunity Shops took some items and the rest, two large furniture vans full, was transported to large units in a storage depot in Ivanhoe.

Bev and I moved into the small dwelling in Viewbank and started to look for a new home. Having found a suitable residence at 14 Erinne Court, St. Helena we moved in in gentle stages. Once the storage units were empty, we sold the Viewbank property took a deep breath and relaxed. In all the process took about eight months and was all-consuming and best forgotten.

~~~

Retirement has been, and continues to be, a time of great joy. It has been filled with interest, completely different to medical matters which dominated my working life. There have been projects which have enabled me to make a worthwhile contribution to the community.

Bev and I have been fortunate to develop many new friendships while continuing the relationships we had developed with other people in earlier years.

REFLECTION

A Fortunate Life is a classic piece of Australian literature, an autobiography written by Albert Facey and published when he was 87 years old. It resonates with me as, although my life has been very different to that of Facey, I believe that I too have had a fortunate life.

I was fortunate to be born into and raised in a conservative, middle-class, religious family which expounded the principles of fairness and respect for others; and to receive my primary and secondary education in schools which had similar ideals. I was fortunate to have good role models, particularly my parents, but also teachers at Carey and members of the Coburg Baptist Church community.

I was fortunate to realise at an early age that my career lay in the medical profession and to be able to receive undergraduate training at Melbourne University. After exposure to many branches of medicine during the first three years of postgraduate training I realised that obstetrics and gynaecology, the care of women, was the one I enjoyed most and was fortunate to be able to pursue that speciality during three and a half years of further training. I was fortunate to enjoy working in this area for the whole of my professional life.

I was fortunate to meet Bev early in our lives and for us to form a successful life-long partnership. Bev has been extremely busy as the linchpin of our relationship producing four children in six years and raising them with minimal interference and without a great deal of help from me. In similar vein she has organised the various homes we have lived in – the final tally is 12 – and their gardens, again with minimal interference. She acted as out-of-hours secretary and relieving receptionist in my consulting rooms. Bev and I are fortunate to have four children and ten grandchildren who are all healthy and have a well-developed work ethic. There is strong bonding between the grandchildren who are as close as siblings.

I was fortunate to be able to pursue many interests outside medicine. Sporting activities have been a joy. Country life was important; I enjoyed developing some of the skills needed to manage a farm property and was delighted to be part of a country town community.

I was fortunate to be able to organise retirement from medical practice gradually over 17 years. I have found retirement to be particularly interesting and rewarding. As well as the various projects with which we have been involved, Bev and I have had more time to devote to our children and grandchildren, to maintain existing friendships and to develop new friendships with a wide range of people.

~~~

One of the highlights of the family celebration held to mark my 80th birthday was a session when, mellow after a formal dinner accompanied by excellent wines and speeches, the grandchildren asked a series of questions regarding various aspects of my life. These questions are worthy of further consideration. Some have been answered, at least in part, in earlier chapters of this book.

Why did you decide to make your career in medicine?

The decision was undoubtedly made because I could see that my father, my most important role model, led an interesting life as a general practitioner and enjoyed his work. Furthermore, I was fascinated by his stories of some of the problems with which he had to deal. The notions of 'wanting to make a difference' or 'helping the sick or injured' or 'entering the medical course because my matriculation results were good enough' were not considerations in making the decision, but the fact that I would always be able to earn a reasonable living certainly was.

What advice do you have for a young person trying to choose their career?

There are many people in the community who do not enjoy their work and who, as a result, are unhappy. With a working life of 40 or 50 years it is extremely important that you avoid this pitfall. It may take some years and several false starts before you find the correct occupation, but it is much better to do the searching for the right job at a young age than to be forced to change later in life or, worse still, to be miserable at work for many years.

Having found the correct occupation, it is important to enter it with gusto and to arrange appropriate training so as to develop the requisite skills even though this may limit your initial remuneration.

Why did you choose to specialise in Obstetrics and Gynaecology?

The decision was an emotional one taken because I enjoyed the work at RWH enormously, despite the large clinical workload. The mix of surgery, procedures in delivery suite and counselling of patients was great, as was the fact that most patients were happy and achieved a good outcome.

What was the most enjoyable part of your work?

I enjoyed all aspects of my work, the clinical care of patients, the providing of information and counselling to patients and the provision of theoretical and practical instruction to nurses, medical students, and doctors in-training. Most enjoyable were gynaecological surgery and being involved in difficult births requiring intervention – twins, breech and forcep deliveries.

What were the most stressful situations you encountered during your career?

There is no debate about this, and the case is described in the section of the book detailing some clinical problems. A patient died on the operating table from a massive amniotic fluid embolism whilst I was performing an elective Caesarean Section for major placenta praevia. Leading the attempted but unsuccessful resuscitation with the anaesthetist then telling the husband that his wife had died was incredibly stressful.

There were, of course, many near misses where appropriate clinical care rescued the patient from a life-threatening situation. The commonest of these were cases of large post-partum haemorrhage (heavy bleeding shortly after birth) which can rapidly become life-threatening and requires immediate appropriate management. This complication is doubly stressful as it occurs suddenly when all seems to be normal and the patient, her partner and the medical and nursing staff are all enjoying the new baby.

How did you cope with drinking alcohol when you were on call most of the time?

I did not become a teetotaller but learned to drink within safe limits so that my ability to function was not impaired. To this end I was encouraged by some of the investigative work that was done before testing for blood alcohol levels was introduced in Victoria in 1976; some investigators showed that people who took one or two standard drinks in one hour performed better behind the wheel of a car than those who had not taken any alcohol – probably because they consciously drove more carefully knowing they had alcohol in their system. Consequently, I limited my alcohol intake to a maximum of two standard drinks in the first hour, then one per hour after that to a total of four. I found this was not a hardship nor did it interfere with my ability to function appropriately.

REFLECTION

What is the secret to being married for 55 years?

In a word, respect! Respect for a person translates to love, care, and support for them. Each partner will bring different skills to the relationship and must be encouraged to use these skills. While having similar goals and sharing similar interests contribute to an efficient and enjoyable partnership it is important that each person has space for, and is encouraged to pursue, their own special interests.

Why do you go to Church?

The simplistic answer is that it is a habit ingrained during my childhood and maintained despite the enormous change in my theology that has occurred during the years. It is more complex than that – I enjoy the peace that accompanies the conventional type of church service with singing of hymns, prayers and a sermon delivered by the minister. More important is the maintenance of close ties with friends who have similar interests and a similar outlook on life.

What were the negative aspects of your career and how did you cope with them?

The major challenges were the long hours on duty with frequent interruption to planned day-time work, to family life and to sleep at night; and having to cope with frequent stressful situations.

A calm personality and a receptionist with good people skills were helpful in coping with interruptions to daytime routine work. Similarly, equanimity and self-confidence were needed to cope with the stressful clinical situations which occurred in the delivery suite and the operating theatre.

In response to the frequent interruptions to sleep I developed the ability to catnap and to function at a reasonable level even when severely sleep deprived.

This skill I retain to this day much to Bev's chagrin when I fall asleep during concerts or films.

Most importantly, I had a life-partner in Bev who understood, and was able to contend with, the interruptions to family life. She had the skills to cope with the children and with the house and garden with minimal help.

I am deeply conscious that Bev and the children were neglected because of the demands of my career and frequently rued that we were, as a family, missing out on many things that other families enjoy. However, I do take comfort from the fact that the four children are all solid citizens who have established themselves in worthwhile careers and are making a significant contribution to the community.

If you were now aged 18 years, would you follow the same career path?

I would certainly attempt to pursue a career in medicine because of the intellectual stimulus it provokes and the opportunity to relate to people and to contribute to society together with the fact that a degree in medicine ensures that one will always be able to find employment and allows one to choose a career in a vast range of different areas. I would not commit to a particular branch of medicine until I had undertaken several years of postgraduate training and been exposed to several different specialties.

It is unlikely that I would pursue a career in obstetrics and gynaecology because, although I have very much enjoyed my involvement in this discipline, the changes that have occurred to the practice of this speciality in recent years make it less interesting and less challenging and therefore less attractive to me. The work that I enjoyed most, the performing of difficult deliveries in the delivery suite has now been almost entirely replaced by Caesarean Section. Much gynaecological surgery is now performed by sub-specialists greatly reducing the range of procedures performed by general gynaecologists.

~ ~ ~

REFLECTION

It is always instructive, after completing a journey, to review the process and to ponder on the positive and negative aspects of the exercise.

Reviewing the 80-year journey detailed in this book, I am comfortable with the conclusion that positive features significantly outnumber negative ones.

It is wonderful to be able to look back on a family life encompassing a 55 year marriage and four children and ten grandchildren who are all healthy and good caring people; to have enjoyed a career which contributed to the health and wellbeing of many women and babies and gave me the opportunity to teach and counsel medical and nursing trainees; and to be enjoying a retirement which has enabled me to make a contribution to organisations such as Nagambie HealthCare, the Probus club of Heidelberg and the Oceania University of Medicine.

Negative aspects of the journey are obvious; the amount of time devoted to medical practice greatly limited the time available for family and social matters. I am reminded of a quote made by Sir William Osler, a famous physician and a founding professor of the John Hopkins Institute in Baltimore, USA: 'Medicine is a jealous mistress, she will be satisfied with nothing less.' Osler also made the statement: 'We are here to add what we can to life, not to get what we can get from life.'

Having completed the 80-year journey successfully I look forward to whatever life offers in the time that remains.